HERBS FOR THE SEVENTIES

Here at last is a remarkably comprehensive and up-to-date factual account of the uses of herbs for healing, health, and beauty.

Under the stress and strain of modern life, we have a population that suffers from over-eating and under-nourishment, and we all know of many households where whole families are victims of some sort of "pill addiction." Therefore, we feel that now is the time for you to explore the possibilities of looking back at Nature and the humble herb as something more than a mere garnish or seasoning. Consider, along with the great doctor of ancient Greece, Hippocrates, the medicinal properties to be found in plants. Investigate the quality of true beauty that begins with a healthy approach to life.

—GARY NULL AND STAFF
The Dell Health Library

HERBS
for the
SEVENTIES

GARY AND STEVE NULL

A DELL BOOK

TO

J.I. Rodale and Staff
Adelle Davis
Carlton Fredericks
Gayelord Hauser
Linda Clark
John Lust
Lelord Kordel
Carlson Wade
Herbert Shelton
Paul C. Bragg
Bob Hoffman
H.E. Kirschner
Linus Pauling
Ralph Nader

Published by
DELL PUBLISHING CO., INC.
1 Dag Hammarskjold Plaza
New York, New York 10017

Reprinted by arrangement with
Robert Speller & Sons, Publishers, Inc.
New York, New York 10010

Printed in the United States of America

First Dell printing—September 1973

TABLE OF CONTENTS

Herbs For The Seventies

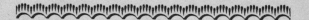

A BRIEF HISTORY

The practice of medical herbalism has probably existed since the emergence of man, but one of the first known cultures recorded to have practiced the use of herbal medicines was the ancient Chinese of some 5,000 years ago.

Upon his death in 2697 B.C., the Emperor Shen Nung was 123 years old. He became known as the Patron God of Agriculture because his life had been spent in the pursuit of the secrets of Nature.

After inventing the plough with which to work the soil, he turned his attention inward to the study of the human body and its reactions to medicines and herbal remedies.

He was said to have swallowed a different herb every day in order to study the effect upon his stomach and system. He discovered many poisonous herbs in this fashion but was able to render them impotent by using specific anti-toxins.

One of his discoveries was that of *Ma-huang*, which was said to be beneficial in the treatment of colds, bronchial spasms and asthmatic attacks. Our modern scientists traced the value of the plant to a substance called *ephedrine* which is now used in prescriptions for pulmonary discomforts and as a decongestant.

We know of Emperor Shen Nung's discoveries because he so thoughtfully kept a record of all his work in a book which is now called *Pen Ts'ao Kang Mu*. The book originally was said to have listed three hundred sixty-five plants of medicinal value such as the rhubarb, mahuang, and many others.

This listing is probably one of the earliest known pharmacopoeia as it was ascribed to the year 2700 B.C. The Chinese thought so much of this first pharmacopoeia that new editions were ordered in the Han dynasty, 25-219 A.D., again between 502 and 556 A.D., again in the Tang dynasty, 618-907 A.D., and a final edition which is still in print, during the Ming dynasty in 1596.

Herbs in the Bible

The Bible makes many references to the use of medicinal herbs. The tree of life in the Garden of Eden was recorded in Genesis to have been put there because the leaves were for healing.

The prophet Ezekiel makes reference to the fruit of the tree as man's meat and the leaves of the tree were for man's medicine.

Moses is recorded to have instructed the Israelites in the use of herbs for the healing of the mind and body in the 104th chapter of Psalms.

These are but a few of the many references to

herbs for healing that are mentioned in the Scriptures. You could undoubtedly find many more.

The ancient Egyptians and Greeks were also responsible for a systematic study of herbs and their uses. Among the ancient practitioners of herbal medicine were Hippocrates, Theophrastus, Pliny, Dioscorides, and Galen.

Hippocrates was the first man who studied and practiced medicine as a way of life. He was a Greek physician who lived from 460 B.C. to 377 B.C.

Over three hundred plants are mentioned in his *Hippocratic* writings and over one third of that list is still considered as valid today.

The Greek philosopher, Theophrastus, who lived from 372 to 287 B.C., made the next valuable contribution to herbal knowledge. He made a more systematic study and classification of plants by writing *History of Plants* where he laid the groundwork for the later herbal therapies.

Dioscoridean Herbal lists such herbs as garlic, myrrh, aloes, mallows, lilies, and roses as herbal remedies as far back as the first century A.D. Dioscorides was a Greek physician to the Roman army in Asia.

Galen, 131 to 200 A.D., was the next man to make a lasting contribution to herbal medicine. He was the author of nearly four hundred works.

Galen followed the precedents set by Hippocrates and used diet, massage, and gentle exercise along with his herbal remedies to treat the sick. He was quite popular in his day, but when he announced his theories of healing and of anatomy to the public, he was considered such a radical that he was forced to leave Rome to avoid persecution. His advanced views were accepted later but not before he had led a very tormented life of hiding and moving from place to place.

The Beginnings of Modern Medicine

Until about 1500 A.D., herbs were the sole source of medicine. Hohemhein was responsible for starting the practice of chemically treating disease.

He burned the books of Hippocrates and Galen believing the human body could be chemically purified. He was the first to consider mercury a medicine.

Modern medicine is a successor of the practices of Hohemhein and his descendants.

The monks were influential in keeping the art of herbology alive. They cultivated herb gardens and experimented with the practice of herbal healing.

The nomad Gypsies of mid-Europe also sustained a knowledge of herbal remedies as they migrated from India to Persia and on to Turkey, Spain, England, and Russia.

They had to rely almost entirely upon the forces of nature for their survival and for life itself. Accompanying their remedies is a great deal of herbal folklore and age-old superstitions. Nonetheless, a number of remedies have survived time and trial to bring us such knowledge as marigold flowers to be used for wounds, mistletoe for nervousness, gentian as a tonic, foxglove, which contains digitalis, as a remedy for heart trouble, and yarrow and coltsfoot for bronchitis.

They discovered a number of herbs could be brewed together to concoct a tonic which would nourish the glands, regulate the manufacture of hormones, and invigorate the circulatory system.

This folk tonic was made by steeping a heaping teaspoonful of either gentian root, skullcap, colombo, rue, valerian, vervain, peppermint, or spearmint in water. The liquid was then strained and used as a hot drink before each meal.

The Gypsies relied upon the woods, the forests, and the trees of nature for their health wherever they went. They believed that nettles were good for the skin, as they are rich in iron which aids and improves the complexion.

As an interest to our laboratories today, the Gypsies also used violet plant to treat tumors and surface cancer.

The Value of the Elder

The Gypsies had a great deal of respect for the elder tree. The elder flowers are beneficial in alleviating the thirst from fever when prepared as a tea. When taken hot, it is a remedy for head colds.

The elderberry, when boiled together with crab apple and blackberry juice, is helpful for coughs and colds.

The Gypsies used elder water as a wash for sore

and tired eyes. The tea is also said to soothe nerves and induce sleep.

A healing ointment is prepared by the Gypsies by cooking fresh elder flowers in home-cured, salt-free lard until all the elder juice is extracted.

Another healing ointment is concocted by stewing the green berries in camphorated oil. If rubbed into the chest and back, it is said to soothe coughs and congestion and also it can be used as a dressing for sprains and burns.

There were many unconscious benefactors of herbal discoveries throughout history. The Indians from the Amazonian rain forests, the arrow poisoners from Africa, and Indians from the Andes were all contributors.

The discovery of quinine can be traced back to the aborigines of South America who used the bark of a Peruvian tree to treat malaria. It took two centuries after the cure of a Spanish viceroy, Count de Chincon, in the year 1638, before scientists were able to extract that one substance from the bark as a valuable treatment for malaria.

Extracts from the oil and seeds of the *Chaulmoogra* tree are still used today to treat leprosy and skin diseases as they were originally used years ago by the natives of Southeast Asia.

The "sacred bark" of the Inca Indians, or *Cascara Sagrada,* is said to be valuable in aiding the relief of chronic constipation.

There was the use of ancient European herbs in America just after the first settlements were established here.

The settlers found that the American Indians were already using herbal teas and wild medicinals. They adopted a few of these usages but mostly continued to practice their herbal knowledge which they brought with them from the Old World.

Many of the herbs that we find in America today which are believed to be wild are actually from those early colonial gardens. They can be traced back to the ancient herbs of the Mediterranean region.

New England's Rarities, a book written by John Josselyn, contains a listing of the European herbs that were introduced to America by the early settlers of the seventeenth century.

What We Learned from the American Indian

The American Indians were knowledgeable in the use of herbs and roots and bark for medicinal purposes. They combined their herbal medicines at times with other methods of treatment such as sweat baths, massage, and special diet or fasting.

Because of their herbal knowledge, they were known to recuperate from battle wounds which many times proved fatal to the white men.

Astringent root was one of their herbal secrets. It was used as a remedy to stop bleeding when the dried root was powdered and put around the open wound and then bandaged. The Indian name for the root is *Hon-Kos-Kao-Ga-Sha.*

Sassafras or *pavame* was a widely used herb

among the American Indians. The powdered sassafras root has been used as a substitute for tea or coffee in the past under the name of *salap* or *saloop*.

The Iroquois prepared a tea from the root-bark. They used this to treat rheumatism, gave it as a tonic after childbirth, and considered it a purifier to the blood. They also administered it as a bladder, kidney and throat remedy for infection and as a tonic for the stomach and bowels.

The Mohawk Indians soaked and strained the pith from the young sassafras shoots to use as an eyewash to reduce inflammation.

When the early settlers first came to the New World they were surprised to find the "primitive" Indians had knowledge of herbal healing. The Indians in fact, relied entirely upon the secrets of Nature for their healing sources. As a result, they roamed the plains of North America and were healthy, vigorous, and prone to long lives.

The early missionaries reported that the Indians' eyesight was unusually strong and free from the problems of squint, blurring, ache, dim vision, and near- and far-sightedness.

The Indians were totally dependent upon Nature and seemed to have been rewarded with magnificent bodies and freedom from the common diseases that were so prevalent with the white men of that day.

The Indian relied upon the floral medicines of the forest not only to relieve eye illnesses but also to strengthen the eyesight.

The Red Man's existence depended upon strong eyesight and vigorous health to withstand the elements of outdoor living, the rough terrain, the severe climate, and the constant struggle to survive in a natural environment.

The Sioux Indians of the Midwest used an eyewash each time before going into battle in order to strengthen their eyesight.

A small golden-flowered plant grew abundantly in the woodlands of the Midwest. This perennial plant has a seal-like scar on its dark yellow root and for this reason is called the golden seal.

The Sioux Indians boiled the golden seal in water and then used it for an eyewash. They believed that it aided in strengthening the eyesight.

Herbalists today also mention golden seal as an eyewash but they suggest adding a small amount of boric acid to the boiling water as well.

The Cheyennes lived along the Platte River and Santa Fe trails and were also noted for their exceptional health and stamina. They had access to a rich and plentiful plant life as a source of medical botany. They favored fennel seed and leaves for their eye-strengthening properties.

Fennel is beneficial for alleviating the aggravations of insect bites, scratches, skin irritations, and visual discomforts. The Cheyenne were aware of the medicinal values of fennel long before the colonists.

An eyewash made from boiling the leaves and/or seeds of fennel in water will soothe and relax tired eyes. It is believed that tension plays an ex-

tensive role in the cause of eye strain and the dim-
inution of eyesight. Relaxation is a key factor in
the Cheyenne's herbal eyewash treatment.

The Nez Percés

Lewis and Clark mentioned the exceptional eye
health and physical vitality of the Nez Percés of
the Northwest. They credited this remarkable eyesight and health to the herbs of Nature.

We learn of the Nez Percés' herbal secrets from
the chronicles and journals of the colonists of the
day. These Indians combined red raspberry leaves
and witch hazel in boiling water, strained the
mixture, and then used it as a wet pack and herbal wash for the eyes.

An herb poultice was used by the Apaches to
heal wounds, lacerations, injuries, and eye inflammation. "The Prescott Miner," a paper of the
1860's, reported that the medicine men of the
Apache tribes made this healing poultice from the
bark of the slippery elm.

The slippery elm herb worked to draw out infectious wastes and to soothe tired, inflamed, itchy,
grainy, and ailing eyes when it was applied as a
poultice for periods of thirty minutes or longer.
The Apaches were credited with superior vision.

The following natural remedies for eye strength
are based upon folklore that is said to have been
practiced among the various tribes of Indians in
North America. The remedies can be a valuable
source of eye refreshment for today.

Tea for the Eyes. The Indians knew about this secret long before it was practiced by our great-grandmothers. To rest and brighten the eyes, herbal tea is used to saturate gauze pads. The gauze pads are then placed onto the eyes while resting in a prone position for thirty minutes.

Green tea can also be used in this fashion. Steep in rose water and apply to the eyes with absorbent cotton pads while resting.

Witch Hazel. The pioneers used witch hazel as an eyewash. Once again the cotton pad method is used while lying down. Refrigerating this solution before using can be an added refreshment to the eyes.

Cherokee Eyewash. The Cherokees used a powder to soothe inflamed, infected, and diseased eyes. It was later discovered that this powder was actually a crude form of boric acid. A small amount of boric acid was said to have been boiled in water and then cooled and used as a soothing eyewash among the Cherokees.

Tea Bags. Wet tea bags are a more modern form of the Indian eyewash. Two wet herbal tea bags can be placed on the eyes while resting for a simple refreshment for tired eyes.

Hot Washcloth. A hot washcloth is an Indian-inspired eye healer. Fold a washcloth into four layers and submerge in hot water. Wring out the excess water and apply to the eyes. A dry towel may be used to cover the cloth to sustain the heat. Repeat as often as necessary for twenty minutes of heat.

Hot to Cold. A thirty-minute application of hot water cloths on the eyes, followed by thirty minutes of cold water, will help soothe nervous eye tremors and to restore some dimming vision.

The effect of alternating water temperatures is that the heat causes expansion and the cold causes contraction, producing a self-cleansing action on visual congestion.

This visual congestion occurs many times from overworking the blood vessels of the eyes or because of the bloodstream becoming viscous as a result of accumulation of too many waste products. Slow, stagnant circulation also causes eye congestion.

Alternating the cold and warm water eye baths either with an eyecup, washcloth, or with just the palms of your hands, helps to clean out infectious wastes and corrosive acids that may have accumulated in the visual arteries and vessels that are impeding healthful sight.

A pinch of salt may be added to warm water when using it as an application for the eyes to help ease tiredness. It is important that all these methods of eyewash be performed while lying in a prone position in order to relax as much as possible.

Poultices. In the case of blocked tear ducts, a poultice can be made from horsetail tea for a soothing effect. Marigold tea and eyebright tea are also good sources for natural eye baths. Charcoal poultices have been used to help soothe eye inflammation when applied at a cool temperature.

More Indian Knowledge

John Lighthall, the author of *The Indian House-hold Medicine Guide,* was born part Indian in the year 1856. He spent thirteen years of his adult life acquainting himself with the Indian medical knowledge of herbs and their various preparations. He was impressed with the fact that the herbal formulas were effective without ever seeming to harm the patients of the medicine men. These are some of the Indian remedies which he passed on in his book in 1883.

A Poplar Tonic

According to Lighthall, there are many valuable properties to be found in the bark of the poplar. He recommended that a tonic could be made of either the white or yellow inner bark of poplar in combination with the inner bark of dogwood and the root of sarsaparilla. This tonic could be used to increase appetite, strengthen nerves, and to restore a natural color to the complexion of convalescents in any cases of general debility accompanied by feeble digestion.

Another Indian formula used to help rheumatism, stimulate appetite, strengthen nerves and purify blood, was made from rattle root, prickly ash bark, poplar bark, sarsaparilla root, dogwood, and wild cherry. Lighthall combined both of the above formulas with "whisky" as a preservative.

Blue Flag

Lighthall reports that the green root is a valuable part of the *Iris versicolor,* or blue flag. He continues that the Indians considered it to be a stimulant for the glandular system and a remedy for blood diseases. They believed, he states, that the tincture promoted excretion and therefore they used it as a treatment for thyroid conditions, scrofula, and other glandular and blood diseases.

Gum, tannin, resinous matter, acid, and starch are all present in blue flag. It has been called an alterative because of its blood purifying compounds, a cathartic, a stimulant, and a diuretic.

European countries used blue flag for skin diseases, certain types of deafness, for ringing in the ears, and also as a thyroid normalizer.

Elecampane

Lighthall wrote in his *Indian Household Medicine Guide* that elecampane was used as a mild, harmless, slow-working tonic by the Indians for the treatment of skin diseases, bronchitis, or any disorders of the mucous linings or lungs in general. A decoction was made of the elecampane root, the spikenard root, and the comfrey root which had to be taken for a long period of time to obtain the desired relief.

Elecampane contains volatile oil, wax, ash, acrid resin, a bitter principle, *helenin,* and is one of Nature's richest sources of inulin. Helenin has been found to be a powerful bactericide and antiseptic because of its alkaloid property.

Elecampane is used in conjunction with other herbs to combat the respiratory disorders of asthma and bronchitis, and the inflammation of the nose and throat.

It is said to help control mucous discharge and excessive cough and is even used in the form of lozenges and syrups for that purpose.

A hot tonic for the relief of coughs is made by mixing elecampane, angelica, comfrey, and spikenard roots with horehound tops and steeping the entire mixture in honey.

Butternut

Lighthall referred to butternut as the "king of constipation." The Indians made a tincture of the inner bark which was gathered in the fall of the year. He claimed that he found it to be the only cathartic that did not result in constipation after its initial relief. In this way, its cathartic action surpasses that of calomel, may apple root, colocynth, jalap, senna, or gamboge, in that it brings a lasting relief.

Butternut is still classified as an excellent laxative today. It contains juglandic acid, volatile oil, tannin, fixed oil, ash, resin, and potassium, plus some calcium, sodium, and aluminum.

It is cited as a cathartic, tonic, and a vermifuge and is used in the form of a tincture, extract, syrup, or pill. It is said to operate without irritation or unpleasant after effects.

Red Clover

Red clover was used primarily as a tea among the Indians to soothe irritations of the general respiratory tract such as asthma, hoarseness, colds, coughs, and all troubles pertaining to the lungs, windpipe, and bronchial tubes.

A strong tea is made from the blossoms, or a cough syrup can be made from the juice of roasted onions, strained honey and the blossoms of red clover.

Sarsaparilla

Lighthall mentions sarsaparilla's medicine value among the Indians. The tincture, or any of various preparations, was made immediately after gathering the root in the months of July and September. The root is alterative in its action and may be used in cases of blood disease and eruptions of the skin. It works as a blood purifier, stimulates the sudoriferous and sebaceous glands, increases the appetite, counteracts constipation, and is mild to the kidneys.

Navajo Indians

Before their introduction to the white man's food, the Navajos were known for the absence of high blood pressure and obesity among their people.

For gout, they made a tonic from the crushed leaves and branches of the *Gaillardia,* a carduaceous herb. These were added to lukewarm water and applied internally and externally.

The Navajo remedy for rheumatic stiffness was to prepare a tonic from the leaves and branches of the barberry bush.

Watercress was used as a tonic after giving birth. To assist with the delivery, greasewood and sage brush were used.

Snuff was prepared from gentian to use for headache and nose trouble. Blue-eyed grass, aster, and milkweed were also used for nose trouble.

Red juniper and *te'ole* grass were rubbed into the hair for dandruff, and fresh green camphor leaves or pitch from piñon trees were placed on wounds or cuts as a cure.

Contemporary Herbalists

Some of the most prominent of the early practitioners of herbology were Gerard, Parkinson, and Culpeper. An Englishman, Gerard was best known for his work entitled *The Herball or General Historie of Plants* which was published in 1597.

The King's herbalist and director of the Royal Gardens, John Parkinson (1567-1650), divided a garden into four parts, following the tradition of the ancient Persians: the Garden of Flowers, the Kitchen Garden, the Orchard, and the healing herbs or Simples, as it was called. He was responsible for *Paradisus Terrestris,* published in 1629, and *Theatrum Botanicum,* published in 1640.

Nicholas Culpeper

The most popular name to be associated with herbal practice is that of Nicholas Culpeper, 1616-1654. He is known as the Father of English Herbology and also as a student of astrology. He believed that the stars of the universe had an important effect upon the herbs and upon man. He associated a different planet to each herb and to each disease. He then used these associations when evaluating a patient's illness.

One of his books, *the Complete Herbal* which was first published over three hundred years ago, is still in demand today.

Other Contemporaries

Other important names synonymous with the development of modern medical herbalism are Samuel Thomson (1769-1843), A. I. Coffin (1798-1866), Samuel Westcotte Tilke (born 1794), and John Skelton. Each of these men played a vital role in researching, experimenting, and recording the use of herbs for medicinal purposes. Each man helped to stress the importance of food in the causation of disease or the lack of good health.

To quote one of the modern naturalists, J. R.

Bulfairo, ". . . And so has it been through history: Man's ultimate conquest to emerge from the frailties of our existence into a healthier way of life by the use of Nature's bountiful cornucopia."

THE "HERB WAY FOR THE 70's"

*Only as far as the masters of the world have
called in Nature to their aid, can they reach
the height of magnificence . . .* —RALPH
WALDO EMERSON

Nature has provided mankind with remedies for
every disease that might afflict him, and possibly
no other source of medicinal properties is more
beneficial for our good health than herbs. The
young and old people of today seem to be seeking
a more natural way of living in the midst of noise,
confusion, pollution, overpopulation in city areas,
and mass production in a commercial environment. What better time than this to join with
Emerson and look back to Nature and the humble
herb.

The study of herbs as a science is called by various names other than herbology, such as materia
medica, botany, pharmacology, vegetable drugs, or
pharmacognosy.

Practitioners of the Herbal Way believe that we
are what we eat and what we breathe and how we

use our bodies to exercise the tissues and muscles and joints. They advise that one should pattern one's life after Nature and function as a part of Nature.

All of the other animals know instinctively how to obtain food and healing elements from wild roots, herbs, berries, grasses, and even the flowers of Nature. Only man seems to be ignorant of the wealth to be found in these natural bounties.

The honeybee does not have to be taught that pollen can be used for cleansing. Sick monkeys have not only been observed to have eaten two kinds of herbs for their ailments but have also been seen carrying the herbs to other monkeys who were too sick to hunt for themselves. Even crows and jackdaws, the European crows, which man has tried to poison, have been known to find natural antidotes in sorb berries and mistletoe berries which have saved their lives. They instinctively knew that these berries would induce vomiting and empty their stomachs of the poison. Animals with broken limbs will lie immobile in a ditch or sheltered place until the healing process is completed. From almost the beginning of time, the animals that have roamed the earth have known instinctively where to seek out plants to combat diseases and to nourish their lives.

The herbal knowledge that we do have today has generally come to us from the simple and the primitive; from those who knew nothing of botany or pharmacology but only of Nature and her many secrets in the heart of her roots, stems, barks, juices, leaves, flowers, fruits, seeds, and plants. From generation to generation the information has been handed down to us. Nothing is left for us now but to look and decide for ourselves how much of Nature we will respect.

Hippocrates regarded the physician as only the servant of nature. He wrote that "Nature is the healer of all disease" and believed that herbs are the natural medicines still in Nature's forms. This herbalist's theory goes on to profess that germs are the secondary manifestation of disease and not the primary cause; that we cannot control the fact that we are always in contact with germs. Germs flourish and multiply in the body when conditions are compatible for their survival, therefore it is believed by those such as Hippocrates that we can only control disease to the extent that we can maintain our health in a natural way.

In the practice of materia medica, it is said to be a healthy reaction if the body responds to the intake of unhealthy "food" or poison or deadly fungus by a vigorous and complete emptying of the stomach and the bowels. The better the health, the better the cleansing. Herbal teas are one of the natural remedies which are of assistance to Nature in this throwing-off process. Herbologists maintain that chemically produced medicine will many times stop this natural reaction.

It has been suggested that disease might be looked upon as an effort of Nature to warn you of neglect and to rid the system of conditions that are only a result of the violation of the laws of health; that the cause should be treated or changed rather than just the symptoms as is the case with most chemically prepared drugs. That is to imply that in case of sickness, one should reconsider the habits of eating, sleeping, exercise, elimination, and other health processes. No herbologist is going to guarantee that by taking one herb remedy, a disease is going to be cured in the presence of poor living habits.

What is an Herb?

An herb is defined in the dictionary as a seed plant which does not develop woody persistent tissue, as that of a shrub or tree, but is more or less soft or succulent. The Funk and Wagnalls encyclopedia says that an herb is a botanical term which is applied to any seed plant which does not develop secondary wood in its aboveground parts. The term is applied by pharmacists, it reads, to any plant or plant part which has medicinal properties. Plant parts which are boiled for use as food or seasoning are called culinary herbs or potherbs.

A spice is defined as any of the various vegetable productions which are fragrant or aromatic and pungent to the taste. Thus herbs may be classified as spices as well as herbs. The original classification of plants into herbs, shrubs, and trees goes back to the time of the Greek naturalist Theophrastus.

The first medicines used by mankind were those derived from the vegetable kingdom. Any vegetables appearing on the table are considered as foods today, while any bitter-tasting vegetable is now considered as a medicine. It is almost forgotten that not long ago, bitters were common to the table. They were made from herbs that had ample potash. They were good tonics because they contained potassium, a mineral which is the building cement of muscle and nerve tissue.

Herbs act as astringents, alkalinizers, acidifiers, tonics, diuretics, diaphoretics, laxatives, and serve several other purposes.

THE NERVINES

One class of herbs is known as nervines, or nerve foods. Nervines are mineral foods which supply potash, magnesium, and phosphorus.

Nervines can be divided into two categories: the excitors and the relaxors or depressors. Excitors are the highly acid agents that are low in mineral content. The depressors are more alkaline in nature and tend to conserve or restrict the flow of energy. Inorganic substances high in carbon and low in hydrogen and bromine are depressors. Alcohol is a depressant that relaxes the nerves by starving the tissues and nerves of mineral until the tissues become subject to malnutrition.

Ladies' Slipper

Ladies' slipper is one of the most excellent nervines in the plant kingdom. It is believed to be one of the safest ways to arrest nervous irritability, hysteria, insomnia, and depression. Because it produces no harmful or narcotic effects, it is preferable to certain drugs for quieting the nerves and promoting sleep.

Other Nervine Sources

Organic foods are a source of nerve regeneration and mineral supply. They have a direct effect upon the nerves and tend to assist in maintaining an energy reserve. Foods such as celery, cucumbers, garlic, honey, molasses, red pepper, ginger, and cloves would come under this classification.

The Many Benefits of Celery

Celery was used as a medicine by most of the ancients. It was Hippocrates who first advised over 2400 years ago that celery should be a food as well as a medicine. He also prescribed celery as a diuretic.

It is recorded that celery was a rare item in the England of the seventeenth century and does not seem to have been used as a common vegetable until some two hundred years later. Even today many physicians and nutritionists believe that celery feeds tissues to cleanse, calm, and heal. It is a carminative (expelling and cleansing gas from the alimentary canal), diuretic, tonic, stimulant, emmenagogue, and nervine in its therapeutic action.

Due to its high mineral content and its alkalinity, there are many benefits believed to be acquired by the use of celery in the diet. Each part of the plant has its own particular value, so each should be looked upon separately as a beneficial addition to the diet.

Potassium, sodium, calcium, phosphorus, and iron are to be found in the stalk of celery which is 93.7 percent organic water. One-half cup of diced celery contains more calcium, phosphorus, and vitamin C than an equal amount of raw carrots or nearly twice as much calcium and phosphorus as three leaves of head luttuce. It is of benefit to the nerves if eaten raw. The stalks are also low in calories and will satisfy hunger and relieve a sour stomach.

The leaves of the celery contain vitamins A, B, and C and also potassium, sodium, and an insulin component. Diabetes, acid condition, and gout are helped by this latter ingredient. The crude fiber or cellulose of the leaves is a good source of bulk for aiding regularity of the intestines. Although the leaves contain sulphur acid, their residue is actually a strong alkaline.

The knotty root, or *celeriac*, is also alkaline. It contains potassium, sodium, calcium, iron, silicon, some vitamin A, and is rich in vitamin B. It can be grated to use in salads, soups, or stews. Celeriac is also a source of improvement for nervous conditions and for dropsy.

The concentrated, acid-forming starches that most Americans compulsively consume usually create deposits of insoluble, inorganic calcium in the system and joints. Celery has been investigated as a possible agent for breaking down the inorganic calcium into a solution until at least some of it can be eliminated from the body. This is said to take place because of the organic sodium found in celery. This therapeutic action is of value in the treatment of arthritis, rheumatism, and lumbago.

Raw celery juice can settle the occasional acid stomach because of its alkaline nature. The sodium in celery is a great neutralizer. The raw juice has also been found to be a refresher in hot, dry weather as it has the effect of normalizing the body temperature.

The greener celery known as Pascal is better for nutritional purposes than the whiter product found in some supermarkets today. The whiter the celery, the more it has been bleached, the less it has to offer as a natural source of nutrition.

Iodine in Nervines

The presence of iodine in foods will excite the nerves to contraction and stimulate the cells and tissues by a direct action through the thyroid gland. Ocean foods contain iodine in the best form and are also a fine source of minerals. They are therefore classified as excitors in the nervine family. Dulse and kelp are examples of ocean plants which induce slow assimilation.

Kelp is not only a source of iodine which is essential for the proper functioning of the thyroid, but it is also a source of vitamins A, C, D, B complex, E, and K. It has been known to relieve glandular disturbances which may result in goiter, rickets, eczema, constipation, asthma, neuritis, and low vitality. The professional guides of Tibet carry kelp when climbing to relieve muscle strain, difficult breathing, and as a source of energy. Kelp is also an arterial cleansing agent which gives tone to the walls of the blood vessels and is therefore helpful in some cases of arterial tension or high blood pressure.

Kelp has a normalizing effect upon the reproductive organs, including the uterus, prostate gland, testes, and ovaries.

Kelp can be added to the diet in a number of ways. In its powdered form it can be sprinkled on salads, cottage cheese, soups, fruit juices, or baked potatoes. As a seasoning, it can be used as a salt substitute or it can be added in the baking of bread or cookies.

Watercress for Sunlight Energy

Another source of iodine is the much overlooked watercress. It does not contain the high amount of iodine that is found in kelp and other sea vegetation but it is more valuable as a source of this vital element than other land plants. Ample use of iodine-rich watercress is good Preventive Medicine.

Watercress, like parsley, is usually looked upon as a decorative green, a mere garnish. By treating it as such, we are passing up a valuable source of vitamins C, A, B, G, and E. It contains almost twice as much vitamin C as spinach and also supplies a higher percentage of essential organic minerals than spinach. It has been called the "scurvy grass" because of its vitamin C content which has proved to be helpful in the treatment of scurvy. Its vitamin C element also makes it an admirable food for the elderly for it helps maintain the suppleness of the small blood vessels and thus aids in warding off hardening of the arteries.

The sulphur content of watercress aids in the proper functioning of the glands, particularly the pancreas. It is especially good for building up the blood in some cases of anemia because of the iron, copper, and manganese it contains. Its manganese element is helpful for nourishment of the pituitary glands.

Liberal quantities of this herb are a good addition to the daily diet. It can be used in salads like head lettuce and will prove to be a much richer supply of minerals and vitamin C than that familiar salad green. Watercress is stimulating to the digestion and has a refreshing taste. It goes particularly well with meat because of its fresh, spicy flavor. It can be cooked the same as other popular greens or, of course, as a soup but is most nutritious when eaten raw. An old Italian favorite is to serve watercress as a salad with oil, vinegar, and garlic.

Parsley: Another Valuable "Garnish"

Parsley is another little table garnish which should be eaten rather than thrown away. It contains as much as 22,500 units of vitamin A per ounce which is so necessary for the health of the eyes and optic nerve system. Carrots, which are so highly respected for the prevention of night-blindness, contain only 1,275 units per ounce. The rich amount of vitamin C found in parsley helps to strengthen the body's resistance to infection and to maintain the tissue health of bones, teeth, and gums. It provides four times as much vitamin C as does an equal weight of oranges.

Parsley also ranks high as a source of vitamin B1 and has been recommended as a food for the elderly because of its stimulating influence upon the digestion and its beneficial assistance in keeping the organs of the urinary system in good health. The iron content in parsley far surpasses that of spinach in a ratio of five to one. Parsley is also a good source of manganese and potassium and contains more calcium and phosphorus than most vegetables. In addition to its vitamin and mineral content, parsley is also a source of sugar, mucilage, starch, volatile oil, and apiol.

Parsley has been used as a folk medicine for menstrual irregularities and cramps because of its emmenagogic action, and has been credited since ancient times with having a favorable influence upon the gallbladder, liver, and spleen.

Parsley may be added fresh to salads along with the other greens, or it may be cooked with soups, cabbage or root vegetables. It can be sprinkled into broths, eggs, and vegetable dishes or added to salad dressings, sauces, meat loafs, broiled hamburgers, and fish. It can be used as a stuffing for fowl or dried and made into a tea which is very helpful for urinary trouble and prostate pressure.

Along with watercress, parsley has been considered a Preventive Medicine but at any rate, should be looked upon in the future as more than just a garnish.

ALFALFA IS "PEOPLE" FOOD

Who would ever think that alfalfa. which has been considered a mere cattle fodder and feed for chickens and pigs for years, would turn out to be one of the most valuable sources of nutrition for humans? Who would ever believe that something that costs so little could give you so much in return?

This healing grass has been around for several thousand years. The Arabs used it as an elixir for their horses. They believed that the animals became stronger and more fleet-footed on the desert sands as a result.

The green leaves of this legume contain eight essential enzymes including *lipase,* which splits fats; *amylase,* which works on starches; *coagulase,* which coagulates milk and clots blood; *emulsin,* which works on sugars; *invertase,* which changes cane sugar into dextrose; *peroxidase,* which works as an oxidizer in the blood; *pectinase,* which converts a pectin substance into a vegetable jelly; and *protase,* which digests proteins.

Frank Bower was the man responsible for first

discovering the enzyme properties in alfalfa. He is often referred to as the "Father of Alfalfa." He has tested the use of alfalfa for stomach ailments, gas pains, ulcerous conditions, poor appetite, and many other complaints.

Mr. Bower has reported that in one specific incident, alfalfa tea was used successfully to stimulate the appetite of a man suffering from anemia who had no appetite. Mr. Bower also found alfalfa an excellent diuretic for the kidneys, a good regulator of the bowels, and a rich source of vitamin D, lime, and phosphorus all of which encourage strong bones and teeth in growing children.

He reported that alfalfa tea has proved effective in cases of dropsy and that it is helpful in treating recuperative cases of narcotic and alcoholic addiction. He also used alfalfa in cases of overweight.

There are other reports of alfalfa tea being used successfully to help nourish hormonal channels and to stimulate lazy glands when substituted in place of caffeine-containing coffee and tannic acid-containing tea.

The alfalfa tea has been administered in cases of prostate and bladder difficulties, and for the discomfort of lumbago.

The chlorophyll, enzymes, minerals, and vitamins in alfalfa are an aid to digestion and a source of stimulation for the appetite.

The enzymes are plentiful enough to assist in digesting all four of the classes of food: the proteins, fats, starches, and sugars.

Alfalfa is a prime source of hormone-feeding protein as well as containing vitamin U which is an aid for peptic ulcers.

Some doctors believe that the chlorophyll found in alfalfa has a stimulating effect upon the growth of the supportive connective tissue cells and upon the development of the tissues of granulation. It has been speculated that an effective barrier to bacterial invasion is developed with its presence in the system because of the cell activity.

When the herb is reduced to a powder and mixed with cider vinegar and honey and water, it is used for arthritis.

Alfalfa can be purchased from the health food store in various forms. It is ground into a meal, cultured in sprouters, made into tea, eaten as seeds, taken as tablets or food supplements, found in alfalfa fudge candy, and is available as the organic base in high potency vitamin tablets, or as a dehydrated alfalfa juice.

One of the most palatable forms of this source of nutrition is the alfalfa sprouts. The sprouts of grains and legumes develop liberal quantities of vitamins so that a healthy amount of nutrition can be expected to be found in the alfalfa sprouts.

Seed sprouts are believed to be excellent producers of vitamins A, B-complex, and C. Certain legume sprouts will furnish as much as half of the daily vitamin C requirement in just one serving. Alfalfa sprouts are also a source of vitamins D, E, G, K, and U.

The cell-building amino acids, *arginine, lysine,*

theronine, and *tryptophane,* are found in these sprouts plus organic phosphorus, chlorine, silicon, aluminum, magnesium, sulphur, sodium, and potassium, all in digestible forms.

The sprouts are a prime source of calcium which is needed to stabilize nerves and to help normalize glandular functions. Some tests are said to have shown that one hundred-fifty percent more protein is to be found in alfalfa sprouts than in the grains, wheat and corn. The healing properties of alfalfa sprouts are now thought to be traceable to the chorophyll contents.

The sprouts freshen the taste in the mouth and leave the breath smelling pleasant and sweet. They also encourage regularity in the bowels, stimulate the appetite, and give a feeling of warmth to the stomach.

Alfalfa sprouts have been used to stop tooth decay and generally help to keep the teeth strong because of their rich iron, calcium, and phosphorus content.

Alfalfa sprouts were first recorded as a source of good health in a book written in 2939 B.C. by the Emperor of China.

Hence, we learn a simple lesson from the beasts: that sweet-smelling alfalfa which we've called fodder and feed is really people food, too!

THE LEMON—ANOTHER
OF NATURE'S TREASURES

The everyday lemon is another of Nature's prizes that we usually take for granted in the rush of modern shopping. Its freshness is even overlooked by some in preference to frozen lemon juice, and bottled lemon extract. Unknown to most, this common accent to a cup of tea or a piece of broiled fish is a valuable source of cellular building properties.

The lemon contains calcium, phosphorus, magnesium, potassium and vitamin C. These elements nourish the brain and nerve cells. In addition, vitamin P which is called *citrin*, is found in the white, spongy layer beneath the rind.

The rind contains the oil of lemon which is used in lemon flavorings and in the manufacture of perfumes. Lemon pulp was used at one time in the manufacture of citric acid, and is now used to make concentrated lemon juice.

A native of the Near East, the lemon was first brought to Spain and northern Africa during the Middle Ages. The majority of the commercial U.S. lemons are grown in southern California today, although some also come to us from Florida. The cultivated lemon is a hybrid of two wild species of citrus. Some geneticists believe the lemon is derived from the lime and citron.

The lemon can work as an antiseptic to cleanse the system of impurities and to help prevent sepses or putrefaction. It can serve as a stimulant to the liver by dissolving the uric acid and other poisons in that organ. For liver discomfort, the juice of a lemon has been taken in a glass of hot water before breakfast.

Fresh lemon in a glass of water before each meal will help ease nervous stomach.

Lemon is valuable in soothing diphtheria, asthma, rheumatism, excessive menstruation, heartburn, fevers, and scurvy.

Lemon juice was discovered as a cure for scurvy by a man named Ronssius, some two hundred thirty-one years before it was recognized as the same by the British Navy. Lemon juice was not used as a preventative medicine for scurvy, however, until sixty-nine more years had passed when the English Merchant Marine finally employed it for that purpose.

A daily consumption of lemons was used in some cases of kidney stones to successfully dissolve the urate stones because of the action of the vitamin C it contains.

Fresh, raw lemon juice has been used as an application for external hemorrhoids.

Your grandmother probably knew about using lemon as a bleach for linens. After washing the fabric in lemon juice, it can be hung in the sun to obtain a bleached effect.

Lemon juice can be used to remove food stains and the odors of fish and onion from the hands if applied after washing the dishes.

There are a few simple ways of adding lemons to your everyday diet. The juice can be used as a substitute for vinegar to make your salad dressings more nourishing.

The juice of the lemon may be used as a flavoring for green vegetables, soups, and fruit drinks.

Lemon juice is a tasty way of marinating meat or fish although some nutritionists will not recommend mixing an acid fruit with a protein food as they believe it is difficult on the digestion.

So once again, perhaps we will think twice and take another look at Nature with a little more respect when we take those next three lemons off the grocery shelf.

THE MANY BENEFITS
OF LICORICE

Licorice, or liquorice, as spelled in the old English Herbals, is easily one of the oldest remedies for the complaints of coughs and chest pains. This medicinal herb is even mentioned in hieroglyphics and the ancient clay tablets of Mesopotamia as a medicine and elixir of life.

A generous supply of licorice root is reported to have been buried with the Egyptian king, Tutankhamen, in 1344 B.C. to aid him on his last difficult journey.

For centuries, licorice has been used to treat consumption, dry cough, hoarseness, wheezing and breathlessness, dropsy, constipation, and other discomforts. A record of this "black magic" herb has been found as early as the Hammurabi reign of Babylonia in 1792-1750 B.C. where it is mentioned as a curative agent for respiratory ailments.

The pharaohs of Egypt drank licorice water or mai sus, as they called it. The mai sus was prepared by dropping dried licorice roots into jars of drinking water.

The fame of licorice spread from Mesopotamia

to Greece and other Mediterranean countries. The virtues of licorice as a thirst quencher, a healer, and as a "sweet root" useful for treating asthma and dry cough, were mentioned by Theophrastus, the Greek botanist, several centuries before the birth of Christ.

Licorice root is said to have been carried into battle as a source of first aid by the warriors of Alexander the Great. It was also used during the Roman military campaigns.

The ancient Chinese consumed licorice to increase endurance, encourage supple bodies, and to prolong youthfulness. It was used in the Buddhist ceremonies as a sacred herb. The Chinese herbalist doctors regarded licorice as a potent, curative agent.

Licorice was very popular among the Europeans during the Dark Ages and the centuries to follow. It was introduced in America by the early English settlers where it remained popular even among the Indians.

Dr. Culpeper makes reference to licorice as the "great sweetener of the blood" in his *Complete Herbal* writings. He recommended licorice root boiled with maidenhair and figs as a remedy for dry cough, hoarseness, wheezing, shortness of breath, and pains of the breast and lungs. He considered it a cleansing agent and balsamic because of its soothing action. He believed it could be used as a pectoral, a laxative, and a purgative.

Culpeper recommended the use of a strong decoction of the root and also the extract. He considered the juice of the root to be most effective and mentioned that it is sweeter and better tasting than the root itself.

A member of the pea family, licorice is widely used today as a flavoring for confections and as an emollient and demulcent in medicine. It is also used in fire extinguishers as a foam stabilizer.

The sweetening agent found in licorice roots which is known as *glycyrrhizin,* is the property used in the manufacture of confections and pharmaceutical commodities. It has fifty times the saccharinity of cane sugar although it is said to have never been completely analyzed nor synthetically duplicated. The sweetness is so potent that it is still found to be detectable even when diluted in water as much as twenty thousand times its own strength.

THE MISTLETOE MYSTERY

The use of mistletoe during the Christmas season, like holly and ivy, has lost its meaning in this modern day. There was originally a mystic association with the plant. During the time of the Gauls, the Druid priests considered the presence of mistletoe growing in an oak tree as a divine gift. A ritual was performed annually by the priests to remove the plant or "gift" from the boughs of the sacred oak. The pieces were then divided and cherished as charms or sacred relics and used in remedies for disease. It was also used to induce vomiting in the case of poisoning. The Christmas custom of kissing under the mistletoe originated during this period when the plant was regarded as sacred.

Mistletoe is mentioned in Norse mythology where a branch of it was said to have slain the god, Baldur. Scandinavian legends considered mistletoe a symbol of life and resurrection probably because of its green leaves which wound around bare, winter trees giving the appearance of new life and foliage.

The Persians used mistletoe as far back as 3,000 B.C. as a remedy for epilepsy according to some sources. It was used as a treatment for circulatory and nervous disorders all through history. Hippocrates wrote of the value of mistletoe in the treatment of the spleen as it was also mentioned by Culpeper for the "falling sickness." Sir John Colbatch cited mistletoe as a treatment of epilepsy in 1770 while some French researchers were considering it as a favorable decoction for epilepsy, nervous maladies, convulsions, irritations, and as a toner for the nerves, as far back as 1682.

It was not until 1907 that mistletoe again gained the attention of the medical world, when René Gaultier studied the plant and discovered what he thought to be anti-hemorrhagic properties in mistletoe.

What We Know About Mistletoe Today

Viscum album, or European mistletoe, is the variety of plant thought most beneficial today. It obtains its nourishment in a half-parasitic fashion by attaching itself to such trees as the apple and the poplar. Its botanical name is a Latin derivative meaning "birdlime" which is a sticky substance found as a formation in leaves, berries, and stalks.

The American variety of mistletoe is not considered as decorative as the English and has even been found to be harmful to the trees upon which it attaches itself. It is known as *Phoradendron flavescens,* or *false mistletoe,* and is also half-parasitic.

Mistletoe has been shown to contain choline and acetyl-cholinetyramine substances which are used for the regulation of high blood pressure and circulatory disorders. It also embodies twice the amount of potash and five times as much phosphoric acid in its wood as has been found in its patron tree. The use of mistletoe for medicinal purposes is widely known in Germany even today.

The non-toxic action of Viscum album is thought to be beneficial in the treatment of arteriosclerosis and high blood pressure. Some of the manifestations of high blood pressure in arteriosclerosis are headaches, vomiting, sight disturbances, and a buzzing sound in the ears which are improved by the use of mistletoe because of its tendency to decrease the blood pressure and tone the heart muscle.

There is often an increase in blood pressure during menopause which can cause palpitation, tachycardia, suffocation, and abnormalities in the peripheral circulation. Viscum album has been used as a tonic to help combat these discomforts and for certain uterine complications.

Because of the work of Gaultier and Chobard, mistletoe has been employed as an anti-hemorrhagic in cases of hemorrhages postpartum, epitaxis, tuberculous hemoptysis, and intestinal hemorrhages which have occurred during typhoid fever.

Mistletoe has been used in the treatment of chronic nephritis when patients are suffering from retention of nitrogen. Fresh extract from mistletoe has been combined with hawthorn and wild leek to combat hardening of the arteries and high blood pressure. This method has been employed in conjunction with the elimination of salt and protein from the diet.

Mistletoe extract, or "Visca-drops," has been administered as a deterrent for dizziness of headaches, spells of vertigo, cold feet, and the "pins and needles" of poor circulation in the extremities. "Visca-drops" have been used in conjunction with heart remedies to help in the relief of palpitations, vascular spasms, difficult breathing, and nightly asthma attacks. Homeopathic injections of mistletoe have even been given by some doctors to relieve pains in the joints due to chronic arthritis.

An infusion of mistletoe, *valerian root,* and vervain has been made as a possible remedy to improve a weakened and disordered state of the nervous system. It has a sedative effect upon the solar plexus without having any dangerous side effects and without being habit-forming.

NETTLE—A USELESS WEED OR A USEFUL PLANT?

"In Scotland, I have eaten Nettles, I have slept in Nettle sheets, and I have dined off a Nettle table-cloth. The young and tender Nettle is an excellent potherb. The stalks of the old Nettle are as good as flax for making cloth. I have heard my mother say that she thought Nettle cloth more durable than any species of linen." Thus wrote the Scottish poet Thomas Campbell.

Victor Hugo paid tribute to the herb in *Les Misérables* when he wrote, ". . . When the Nettle is young, its leaf forms an excellent vegetable . . . Chopped, the Nettle is good for poultry, pounded it is good for cattle . . . The seeds mingled with fodder impart a gloss to animals."

Most people who are ignorant of the nettle's worth have considered the plant a nuisance because of its weed-like growth and an undesirable irritation that is caused by the stinging hairs that cover the plant.

Known as the Stinging Nettle, country people usually looked for the Yellow Dock growing near a cluster of nettle for an antidote for the rash.

The leaves of the Yellow Dock can be crushed and applied as a poultice to soothe the burning itch. What most people are not aware of is the fact that the juice of the nettle leaves will cure its own sting.

It is an age-old practice to prepare nettle fibre for the production of linen and thread. The plant was even used to obtain several dyes at one time. Nettle has also been used in paper manufacturing.

Nettles contain calcium, iron, potassium, sodium, and sulphur. Boiling will render the stinging hairs harmless. The dried herb has been used medicinally as a tea for fever, colds, to increase the menstrual flow, for diarrhea, dysentery, piles, hemorrhages, hemorrhoids, gravel, inflammation of the kidneys, and to clean out the urinary canal. Nettle bear is made in England where it is taken by the aged for ailments. German soldiers drank mild nettle tea with sugar as a substitute for coffee and oriental tea.

The dried leaves have been burned and the smoke inhaled for the relief of asthma, according to some folk healers. Gerard mentioned the use of nettles for this purpose. A healing ointment was prepared by the Romans by steeping the leaves in oil. It is used for toothache and sciatica in Russia, and the fresh juice is dropped into open wounds in Jamaica. It was a popular remedy with the Indians for urinary difficulties and excess bleeding.

The bruised leaves have been used to rub onto the skin for the relief of chronic rheumatism, especially by the country people of Germany and Russia.

The presence of potash, tannin, and formic and gallic acid in the nettle's content has worked as an astringent action when given as a dose internally. Nettle juice administered in this way arrests bleeding in cases of nose, lung, and uterine hemorrhages.

Nettles have been used for the relief of constipation. The young spring nettles can be boiled in milk and taken in the mornings upon rising. This remedy has been used to stop migraine headache when it is associated with bilious vomiting. Nettles are a good purifier of the blood.

It is possible for hives to result due to the existence of impure blood and a disordered condition of the stomach and the bowels. A skin rash will appear, accompanied by painful itching or tingling. A folk remedy has been suggested for this condition which includes the use of the nettle. The juice of the nettles is taken internally and the body washed with water and marshmallow soap. This remedy, as with all of the remedies cited in this book, should only be administered under the guiding eye of a qualified physician as the bowels may have a radical reaction to the nettle dosage in this case.

The use of nettles as a medicinal herb is also well known in India and Pakistan. The drug-yielding plants are still generally used in their crude forms in these countries today. In addition to some of the remedial uses already cited, the people of these two countries also employ the use of nettles as an anthelmintic (to expel worms), and for the treatment of jaundice and consumption. The seeds are classified there as diuretic, astringent, and tonic.

There are a number of ways in which to add nettles to the diet. The young leaves can be finely chopped and used as a garnish on soup. The juice can be mixed with other vegetables or with potatoes or with oatmeal soup. To serve with baked or mashed potatoes, the young nettles can be stewed in oil with chopped onions.

Nettle spinach is a palatable dish. The leaves of the stinging nettle plant cook quickly and make an excellent green vegetable addition to the table. Simply cook the leaves in boiling water until tender, then drain. Rinse in hot water twice, season to taste, and serve.

When a plant is looked upon so favorably in so many parts of the world, perhaps it's an indication that we should take another look at its possibilities right here at home. Nature is still the one thing that is consistent in this time of change. Perhaps only within the secrets of Nature can we find the true antidotes for our neglected bodies and our over-pressured minds.

THE OLIVE TREE
—A SYMBOL OF PEACE

Olive trees were first introduced to the New World by the Franciscan Fathers in 1769 near San Diego, California. They were grown by the Egyptians over four thousand years ago. Eight of the original olive trees of the Garden of Gethsemane are still believed to be in existence.

Green olive branches are almost universally considered an emblem of peace as they were among the Greeks, ages ago. The oil is medicinally thought to bring "peace" to those suffering from certain pains and tensions.

Olive Oil

A valuable source of food oil, olive oil contains sixty percent fat. It is rich in potassium which makes it a good cleansing and healing agent. It is also a good source of sodium and calcium. Olive oil is soothing to the digestive tract and can be used both externally and internally for various treatments when it is in its pure form. Much of the olive oil sold commercially is diluted or adulterated with cottonseed oil which renders it less valuable.

The pure oil is used for culinary purposes, salad dressings, cosmetics, soaps, and cleansing solutions. It is also found in liniments, pills, sunburn lotions, plasters and ointments.

Many people suffering from ulcers have found that swallowing a small amount of olive oil before meals eases the digestion and lessens after meal discomfort.

Olive oil has been substituted for the cream in some ulcer diets. It has been found to reduce stomach acids, and because it is unsaturated, it will not raise the blood cholesterol.

Scientific tests have been made to establish the relationship of olive oil to a healthy heart. A very low rate of heart and artery disorder exists among the middle-aged men of Greece where olive oil plays an important part in the diet. Olive oil has also been used successfully to reduce blood cholesterol when used exclusively over all other oils and fats.

Olive oil has been known for ages as a mild and effective laxative even for the very young.

Experiments have been conducted with white mice which have shown that the use of olive oil in the diet seemed to protect the liver, kidneys, and lungs, as well as skin and hair from the adverse effects of X-ray exposures.

These experiments are still being conducted to establish their value in human application.

When the gallbladder, which stores and concentrates bile (the yellow fluid secreted by the liver into the intestinal tract), does not contract enough to completely empty itself, the bile accumulates and eventually creates gallstones.

Olive oil is a good gallbladder tonic as it causes contractions of the gallbladder so that it can empty in a natural way. Olive oil has been found to stimulate bile secretion and absorb fatty acids.

The fresh flowers of St. John's Wort can be infused in olive oil for an herbal application for wounds, sores, swellings, and abrasions.

Olive oil can be combined with glycerin and distilled witch hazel for the relief of painful sunburn.

Warm olive oil has been used as a first aid measure to help remove foreign particles such as grit, ashes, or dirt from the eyes.

An emulsion of olive oil, malted milk, and hot water has been used by those suffering from malnutrition, nervous debility, and constipation.

It may be that this symbol of peace, the olive tree, will also be a source of "peace" for the system if we seek out its medicinal and nutritional potential in the 70's.

ROSEMARY, SAGE AND TIME

Rosemary, a member of the mint family, comes to our table in the 70's with a traditional background. Even Shakespeare was one of the poets who made frequent allusions to its tradition of strengthening the memory. The Romans and Greeks used rosemary as incense in their religious ceremonies and made garlands from the leaves to honor heroes of the day. They even used the herb when embalming the dead as they believed it was symbolic of the soul's immortality.

It has been customary in various parts of the world in past years to include rosemary in bridal wreaths to signify the fond memories the bride would cherish of those she left behind. The herb has even been a mystical symbol of love and loyalty and carried the promise of strengthening the heart as well as the memory.

Rosemary was a part of Christmas decoration at one time in history as it was thought to be a symbol of peace and good will.

The early monks cultivated rosemary for medicinal purposes. They mixed the young tops, leaves, and flowers to brew a tea for nervousness, convulsions, liver trouble, headache, and stomach disorders. For relief of bronchitis and asthma, they mixed the tea with honey. A liniment prepared from rosemary was used for rheumatism and gout.

Culpeper mentions rosemary in his writings as an aid for dizziness, weak eyes, weak memory, gaseous stomach, and indigestion. The Balkans used a solution made from rosemary as a folk remedy for the relief of bone and joint pains. Rosemary is also one of the ingredients in an herbal formula to relieve the pain of migraine headache.

Rosemary tea has been recommended by some herbalists as a remedy for the congestion of colds in the fall and spring.

Throughout history, rosemary has repeatedly been mentioned as an excellent stomachic, meaning it is believed to give strength and tone to the stomach, stimulate the appetite, and aid in digestion.

Rosemary may be added to veal, lamb, roast beef, beans, gravies, sauces, poultry, and rice for seasoning. It should always be added within the last hour of cooking time, as prolonged cooking destroys the flavor.

Sage: Another Traditional Herb

Sage, as a medicinal herb, is mentioned in the writings of Theophrastus, Pliny, and Hippocrates. It was one of the folk remedies associated with the treatment of the spleen. At one time in history, it was known as a sacred herb capable of increasing the life span and rejuvenating the eyes, brain, and glands.

Sage was mentioned in the writings of Gerard as an herb that would encourage alertness and the retention of memory, improve strength, or could be used as a restorative from the effects of palsy. Gerard mentions the use of sage for "night sweats of tuberculosis" and as an aid to digestion after a heavy meal. In his writings, sage flowers were mixed with cinnamon and brandy as a cordial for cardiacs.

Sage has been used by the primitive natives of Africa as a successful poultice for swollen throat glands and tongue when used in accompaniment with a sage gargle.

Sage has been found to be effective in relieving mental exhaustion because of its action on the cortex of the brain. In this way, it strengthened the ability to concentrate.

In cases of general hypersensitivity, sage works as a relaxer.

When taken hot, the infusion stimulates perspiration and when taken cold it is an active diuretic.

A concoction of sage leaves, hot malt vinegar, and water has been used by some medical herbalists for the treatment of fevers, tonsilitis, quinsy, and ulceration of the mouth and throat. The solution was taken internally and used as a gargle thus utilizing its tonic ability.

Some preparations made with sage are used to

check the excessive flow of saliva and to treat bleeding gums.

Sage Seeds, or Chia

The seeds found in some varieties of the sage were considered valuable food to the Indians of Arizona, California, Nevada, New Mexico, and Mexico. These *chia* were considered a source of energy and endurance especially against the effects of the desert heat.

The use of the seeds as a therapeutic medicine has been traced back to the time of Montezuma II where the chia were of such value that they were even accepted as payment for taxes.

Chia was toasted by some Indians and used as a cereal by Mexican natives.

The chia seeds are abundantly rich in potassium, copper, calcium, phosphorus, iron, magnesium, iodine, vitamin B complex, protein, and vitamins E and D.

To add chia seeds to the daily diet they are usually soaked before using or ground into a powder which can be sprinkled over salads, into salad dressings, added to soup, cottage cheese, eggs, mixed with butter or margarine, used in batters such as pancakes, added to yogurt, or employed in any other number of ways.

With all herbal or natural methods of remedy, the importance of perseverance is always stressed. There are no "quick" cures among Nature's secrets; time is always said to be of essence.

THE "MAN-SHAPED" ROOTS

The two medicinal herbs, ginseng and mandrake, can be traced back to ancient Chinese folklore. The roots are considered the valuable part of the plants and can be described as "man-shaped." The Chinese followed a very precise ritual when harvesting the roots. Their medicinal value was only thought to be insured if the roots were dug out at midnight of a full moon in a very specific way. In spite of all the mystical association with these strange roots with their fleshy "arms and legs" and knotty "faces," their medicinal properties are not to be overlooked even today.

Ginseng

The ginseng root has been considered worth its weight in silver and five times its weight in gold at different times in history. The plant had to be protected from extinction by special decree during the reign of Tao Kuang, 1821-1851, because people of the kingdom became so eager to possess it.

Ginseng root or Jen shen, as known by the Chinese, has been an important article of export for China for nearly two hundred years.

American Ginseng vs. Chinese Ginseng

The ginseng that grows wild in the United States is considered to be more valuable among the Chinese than the ginseng that is cultivated in America. It was not until 1905 that the Americans began to credit ginseng with any medical value, although large quantities have been exported to China for that purpose for some time. The early colonists chewed ginseng as a tobacco substitute, and swallowed the juice to ease the stomach.

According to the Chinese, the American ginseng is unlike the Chinese ginseng although the untrained eye could not discern the difference. Chemical analyses have shown that they have practically the same properties and certainly the fact that the Chinese continue to accept the American export as satisfactory would indicate that it must be so.

Both Chinese and American varieties of ginseng contain resin, a saponin, starch, tannin, aromatic bitters, volatile oils, and traces of panacin. The root's healing powers are thought to be attributed to the panacin content.

Ginseng is bitter upon first taste but turns sweet because of its starch properties. Some researchers believe that ginseng's therapeutic value is due to its "non-specific action."

Ginseng has been recommended in cases of anemia, asthma, depression, dizzy spells, exhaustion, headaches, indigestion, insomnia, nausea, nervous disorders, and vascular cramps among others.

It is said that ginseng should never be prepared in metal vessels. It should be stored in crockery except in some rare cases, when it may be left in silver containers.

Ginseng may be cooked in water and the sediment saved to prepare an essence.

Ginseng has been powdered and dissolved in the white of an egg as a Chinese remedy to stimulate the digestion.

A Chinese tonic used to strengthen the heart and avert depression is made by blending pulverized ginseng with lard and dissolving the mixture in wine.

A light broth of ginseng and bamboo leaves is said to be a Chinese sedative.

Raw, minced ginseng has been given as a restorative to weak children.

The Chinese mixed ginseng potion with honey and cinnamon to stimulate blood circulation.

A strong ginseng brew is given as a stimulant after childbirth according to Chinese folk remedies.

An extract can be made from chopped ginseng and orange peel and fortified with honey as a possible remedy for insomnia.

A folk remedy for stiff joints is prepared from the extract of ginseng and rubber tree which must be taken on an empty stomach.

To induce perspiration in times of fever, ginseng can be boiled in water until reduced to half the original amount and then the remains can be amended with a small amount of spring or well water.

Chinese folk remedies also include preparations for urinary difficulties, shortness of breath, headache, swollen eyes, cold hands and feet, a restorative, and to treat kidneys that have suffered the ill effects of cold and dampness.

Mandrake Through the Ages

This simple little plant, whose leaves are eaten by some varieties of bears after winter hibernation to renew vitality, has a long and varied reputation throughout the pages of history. A supply of over twenty books can be found on the subject which were written between 1510 and 1850.

Hippocrates wrote about mandrake in 400 B.C. He believed that it had the medicinal power to relieve depression and anxiety. The surgeons of his day are recorded to have used mandrake as an anesthetic because they believed it contained some mysterious alkali foreign to their knowledge.

Dioscorises makes reference to the anesthetic properties of mandrake in his writings. He believed that if it were administered before an operation, the surgeon could painlessly "cut or cauterize" without waking the drugged patient. There are records to show that mandrake has been used as an anesthetic for surgery for some 2,000 years before the discovery of ether.

History makes note of the mandrake's power as an anesthesia in ancient Jerusalem. While the Romans were busy crucifying the criminals of the day in Palestine, the local women were just as busy administering mandrake-soaked sponges to the victims. Upon taking the juice, the grateful recipients would become insensible as if dead and the Roman soldiers would then remove them from their crosses and return the bodies to their relatives.

There was such a great number of recoveries because of this practice that the Roman governors counterattacked by ordering the bodies to be mutilated before returning them to their homes.

Some people are familiar with legends that associate the mandrake with the sexual orgies of old. These ancient beliefs were derived from the nature of the root of the plant which is said to symbolize a "potent male."

The root is thickish and somewhat tuberous and is forked into two leg-like branches. The reasoning behind this botanical imagery of the ancients was that if the gods chose to make a plant to resemble a man, certainly the plant must possess some power of masculine virility.

The women of the Near East valued the plant for hundreds of years and would gather or purchase it at high prices to hang in their homes. The root of the mandrake was particularly precious to barren women who thought that its presence in the house was a guarantee for conception.

The Bible makes mention of the mandrake as a source of fertility in the thirteenth chapter of Genesis. Rachel, who was barren and childless, pleaded to her happily married sister, "Give me, I pray thee, of thy son's mandrake."

Aphrodisiac?

The small, berry-like yellow fruit of the mandrake, or devil's apple as it was known in Arabia, was also believed to possess secret powers of sexuality. The berries were considered quite a delicacy and a source of sexual prowess.

The mandrake is not an aphrodisiac but you would not have been able to convince a Roman of ancient times of that fact. He always had plenty of mandrake on hand for his orgies.

Even Shakespeare alluded to its reputation in *Henry IV* when one of his characters was referred to as "lecherous as a monkey and the whores called him mandrake." Mandrake is truly the victim of a disreputable past.

There are two varieties of mandrake that are considered useful for medicinal purposes.

The English mandrake is said to have a cathartic and hydrogogue action. It has been used to treat coughs, influenza, bronchitis, the cardiac disorders resulting from rheumatism and gout, and as a treatment in the cases of malarial and zymotic diseases.

The American mandrake is quite different from

the English variety. It is more commonly recognized for its treatment of chronic liver and uterine disorders when combined with senna leaves. It is beneficial for normalizing the function of the glands. It is one of the most potent herbal remedies and should never be administered without the advice of a competent physician.

The Swiss use mandrake to cleanse toxic wastes from the bloodstream. They mix a small amount in a glass of cold water and follow this with a glass of warm water at bedtime.

Ginseng and mandrake are two other possibilities to explore in Nature's book of wonders.

THE MODEST ONION

The onion is one of the oldest vegetables believed to be known to man. Ancient Hebrew and Sanskrit literature even make reference to the cultivation of this simple plant. To the Egyptians it represented a symbol of the entire universe because of its many delicate layers which envelop the bulb. It was associated with the godly in ancient Egypt and actually considered a delicacy among the deities of "Pelusium." In the records of Pliny it was written that "the Onions and Garlic are among the Gods of Egypt, and by these they make their oaths." The Egyptian priests abstained from the use of onions as a food, probably as an ascetic act of self-denial. The common people of the day were said to have held the priests in awe because the nature of this particular sacrifice was considered so great. Who would think that our modest onion of today came from such a grandiose background?

The Romans considered the sea onion a "heart tonic" and a treatment for dropsy as far back as the first century of our era. By referring to the onion as a "heart tonic," the Romans were innocently making the connection between dropsy, fundamental heart irregularity, and digitalis. They were some eighteen hundred years ahead of the medical profession in England in making that "discovery."

The sea onion worked in the case of dropsy because it acted as a diuretic by ridding the body of accumulated liquids. What the Romans did not realize was that it functioned in this favorable way because of its action on the heart which is very much like the action of digitalis. Thus by simply referring to the sea onion as a "heart tonic" and by using it as a treatment for dropsy, they were making a discovery that did not actually become known until early in the nineteenth century.

There are many historical records of the wide use of the sea onion for the treatment of fundamental heart irregularities before the discovery of digitalis. Its action on the heart is so close to that of digitalis that it was not passed in popularity for that remedy until the time of the United States Revolution. It was during this period that Dr. Withering of Birmingham, Alabama, made his discoveries of the digitalis-like action of foxglove. The sea onion is considered one of the oldest sources of digitalis-like action on the heart.

This valuable property of the sea onion can only be found in its bulb. When fresh, the bulb may weigh four to seven pounds but only a small portion of it can be used for this medicinal purpose. The outer coating of the bulb is a parchment-like exterior giving it a similar appearance to an ordinary garden onion.

The Funk and Wagnalls encyclopedia says that "onion" is the common name applied to any biennial herb of the genus *Allium,* belonging to the lily family, but usually restricted to *A. cepa* which is native to Asia and has been cultivated in the temperate and subtropical regions for thousands of years. The encyclopedia goes on to mention that other plants in this genus *Allium* which are also called onions would include the wild onion, *A. cernuum,* the shallot, *A. ascalonicum,* and the green onion or common leek, *A. porrum.* The shallot and the green onion, which have small bulbs, are both also known as "scallions."

The true onion is a bulbous rooted plant that is recognized by most because of its long, hollow leaves which are thickened near the base of the stem. This onion contains sulphurous, volatile oils which give it its pungent taste. Phosphorus, calcium, magnesium, sulphur, sodium, potassium, iron, starch, and acetic acid are all found in its contents.

The onion is a source of vitamins A, B, C, and some iodine, zinc, and silicon. A substance is also found in onion which stimulates the digestive secretions of the pancreas.

One of the most fascinating varieties of the true onion is the Egyptian onion, or top onion, because of its rare way of reproducing itself. A Medusa-like mass of aerial bulblets forms on the top of the stem. This clump of bulbs eventually weight the stem right into the ground to literally replant it-self.

This interesting potherb is easy to recognize be-cause of its strange appearance. It has a fat hollow stalk and a flowering top but the most outstanding feature is the contorted looking growth of the aerial bulbs near the top of the plant.

The onion bulbs and stems are commonly eaten raw or cooked. They make an excellent seasoning in salads or hot dishes.

If a salt-free diet is beginning to seem monoto-nous, a little chopped onion first browned in pea-nut oil will add a nice flavor to cooked vegetable dishes. Simply add your freshly chopped vege-tables to the skillet where the onion has been browning and cover. Let the vegetables cook for ten or fifteen minutes in their own steam. The re-sult is a tasty, nutritious vegetable dish flavored naturally with onion.

If an onion with a milder taste and less pungent odor is preferred, the yellow Bermuda and white Spanish onions have been recommended. These are among the mildest of the cultivated onions as they are planted in warm areas for winter crops. The varieties planted in the cooler regions are known for their stronger taste.

When onions are used in small amounts they as-sist the digestion and help stimulate the circula-tion. However, if they are eaten to excess, they are not only disagreeable to the digestion but can be harmful to the system as well.

A series of experiments found that the overeating of onions can actually induce anemia. These experiments were found to have the same results with humans as they did with animals.

Onions can be a valuable asset to the diet but like all things, it is suggested that they be eaten in moderation to obtain their most beneficial effects.

Members of the Imperial Council of Agricultural Research in India, in their experiments, found onion poultices to be beneficial in the treatment of inflamed throat and sinus.

Dr. S. S. Nehru, president of the Agriculture-in-India Science Congress led these experiments. Wishing to understand the nature of these discoveries, he continued the investigation by isolating the mashed onion in cellophane and quartz containers so that they would not actually come into contact with the skin they were treating. He found that the medicinal value acting upon the inflammation still existed under these conditions but when the onions were placed in glass, lead, iron, or aluminum, the healing action ceased.

These experiments led Dr. Nehru to the realization that onions radiate an electrical energy which seems to be able to pass through cellophane or quartz but which cannot pass through glass, lead, iron, or aluminum.

The number of years through history that onions were used as a prominent home remedy for coughs and colds in India was never associated with these unusual rays of electrical energy before this time.

Mitogenetic Radiation. Professor Gurwitch, an

electrobiologist of Russia, was another investigator into the peculiar power of the onion. He found some years ago that the onion emits a form of ultraviolet radiation which is called "mitogenetic" radiation. According to his discoveries, these radiations appear to stimulate the general activity of the cells and to produce a rejuvenating effect upon the whole system.

Garlic and ginseng were also said to have been found to emit the same radiation. Other researchers have reported that a similarly charged electrical field is also produced by penicillin.

Remedies Made from Onions

Pimples. Onion poultices are effective in the treatment of pimples on the face. Three peeled onions should be sliced and cooked in shortening until they are just transparent. After they have cooled, they can be wrapped in cheesecloth and applied to the pimples as a poultice. The poultice should remain as long as possible in order that the rich minerals and the high fatty contents of the onion can have a chance to work to sterilize the skin infection.

Other Skin Eruptions. Onions pounded with a mallet can be used as a poultice for ulcers, boils, abscesses, and insect bites.

Protruding Piles. This remedy for protruding piles is reportedly known to some natural healers. Finely chop and grate two cups of green onions to be mixed with wheat flour and fried in animal fat until the mixture becomes a salve. The warm poultice is then spread onto a cloth and applied directly to the affected area just before bedtime. The application should be repeated the following night and in some cases the condition has even been relieved in the period of two days.

Pulped onions when generously salted have been used as a poultice for this condition.

Headaches. A remedy for headaches can be prepared by pulping a couple of onions with salt and olive oil. This mixture can then be spread onto a cloth and applied to the forehead.

Warts. It has been reported that raw onion dipped in salt can be applied regularly to warts to help them disappear.

Sprains. A chopped onion mixed with sugar can be spread onto cloth and applied to sprains to help alleviate the soreness.

Scalding Burns. To draw out the heat from a scalding burn, apply a piece of salted onion to the area of discomfort.

For hundreds of years the onion has been employed for the effective relief of high blood pressure. Its use in the treatment of asthmatic conditions and other respiratory disorders is also recorded. For these maladies a slice of raw onion should be eaten or the fumes inhaled.

Certain aromas were associated with the supernatural during ancient history. Such fragrant botanicals as musk, cloves, and incense were employed to invoke good luck as countercharms against the witchcraft of the day. Aromas were also used to influence conjurations.

Because of its strong penetrating odor, the onion was often used in these rituals of superstition. Slices of onion were suspended or placed in every room of a house to purge and protect it from "evil spirits." At the beginning of each day fresh onion slices had to be distributed and the old ones burned. This was also a practice commonly performed during the epidemics and plagues to prevent contagion.

Dr. Fernie wrote a great deal about the onion in 1897. In his writings, he considered the onion a very sensitive organism which is capable of absorbing infectious and "morbid" matter. He makes reference to a cholera epidemic of his day wherein the only cottage of a northern town whose inhabitants escaped the ravages of the plague, was found to have a net of onions hanging from its walls. Upon inspection, he reports that sanitary inspectors found all of the onions to have been diseased. Because of this amazing ability he believes the onion to possess, he warns against ever eating any onion that shows signs of decay as it may contain disease.

The custom of placing onions around the house as a disease preventative is not an uncommon practice today. These "onion people" believe that the most important step to follow if this practice is to be successful is to put fresh onions out each day and to burn the old. They believe that in this way the onions work as traps to absorb all of the dangerous germs that are present in the house.

All of the followers of this ritual are said to insist that no onion which has been bruised, peeled, or sliced for more than a few hours should be eaten.

And so the onion turns out to be not such a modest and humble herb after all but rather a plant gloriously associated with deities and the supernatural. Let us not forget the valuable discoveries that have been made about the onion when next it crosses the palate.

HERBS AS A TREATMENT FOR POISON IVY, POISON OAK AND INSECT BITES

The American Indians were known to have used an herbal remedy for the prevention or treatment of poison ivy. They used the plant known as the jewel weed, or *Impatiens*. A mash was made of the stems and leaves and the juice was then rubbed onto the skin that was affected. It was also rubbed onto the exposed skin as a preventative.

Crushed garlic has also been used as a treatment for these two poisons. It is placed between two layers of gauze and then applied to the irritated areas for about half an hour.

Leaves of green bean, plantain, dandelion, trees, or grass may be crushed and applied for poison ivy and poison oak infection.

Lobelia, golden seal, myrrh, echinacea, bloodroot, and Solomon's seal are all said to have been used for the treatment of these two poisons.

A strong tea may be made from equal parts of white oak bark and lime water which is said to be very good for poison ivy and poison oak. Soak a bandage in the tea and apply to the affected area. Change the bandage as often as it becomes dry.

Insect Bites

The Navajo Indians were said to have treated insect stings by first chewing dodge weed or greasewood and then placing the pulp on the swelling caused by the sting of ants, wasps, or bees.

Bee or wasp venom is highly toxic to some people and should be immediately treated by a doctor if symptoms of chills, dizziness, fever, heavy perspiration, headache, nausea or vomiting, great thirst, throat or chest constrictions, weakness, rapid pulse, or unconsciousness should occur.

For minor bee stings, fresh onion, garlic, or the juice of a lemon can be used. Honey has also been used for this purpose.

The tincture of marigold flowers has been used to relieve the infection of gnat bites.

There are several insect repellents made from herbs used in different parts of the world. In Africa and India, cajuput oil is used as a repellent.

A decoction of camomile flowers can also be prepared as an insect repellent and used as a wash for the body.

The Australians rub their exposed skin with the bruised leaves of eucalyptus. They mix the eucalyptus oil with glycerin in some cases to obtain the same effect.

A solution can be made from quassia chips and cold water to use as a repellent against gnats. This is also used as a treatment for the effects of the bites.

The oil of Pennyroyal is a good protection

against the bites of mosquitoes, gnats, and similar winged pests.

Lavender, geranium, and citronella oils have all been used as insect repellents.

HERBAL BEAUTY

How many times as a child were you told "Beauty is as Beauty does"? Perhaps there is a way to apply this old adage in our adult lives of the 70's.

As the definition of beauty becomes more the essence of naturalness and less the action of putting or "painting" something on, what better time to take a look at the natural ways of achieving our own personal beauty. Some of these ways have been known to man for eons but have become camouflaged in the chemical approach of commercialism today or have quietly been put aside as something "grandmother always did."

Natural beauty is something that is enhanced by consistent beauty care. For those who would explore the natural sources as a possibility, there are three important stages in beauty care that must be considered for this natural "beauty way."

Inner Insurance

The first step in beauty care is one of the most important. To really be assured of healthy glowing skin, sparkling eyes, and lustrous hair, one must first take an honest, objective look at what is consumed in the diet.

A thorough cleansing of the alimentary tract is essential for that outward glow. Without the intrinsic factor of a diet rich in vitamins and minerals, the skin will tend to be dull and muddy looking.

Herb teas and green, leafy vegetables are an excellent source of such needed vitamins and minerals. The dandelion is considered one of nature's best beauty sources as it is rich in vitamin A. One ounce of dandelion greens contains 7,000 units of vitamin A. A deficiency of this vitamin can be detected by rough, scaly skin.

Dandelion greens also supply an abundance of vitamins B1 and C. Vitamin C is needed to help the blood carry oxygen to the skin cells.

Because of the assortment of alkaline salts, such as calcium, sodium, and potassium, the dandelion is a good purifying agent for the body.

The use of dandelion is also believed to promote a healthy circulation and to cleanse the skin of blemishes, besides strengthening weak arteries and restoring gastric balance after vomiting.

Riboflavin deficiency may be the cause of wrinkles around the lips. Dandelion greens are rich in riboflavin which may aid in reducing large pores and expelling blackheads.

The lack of protein in the diet will increase the aging process of the skin as its absence encourages lines and wrinkles to appear. Salt in the food can be another source of wrinkles as it tends to dry out the skin.

White sugar has a disagreeable influence on the lines of the face. Excessive starches and sugars are harmful as they are acid-forming to the system.

Eating for the Complexion

Fats, starches, pastries, gravies, and highly seasoned foods are all enemies of a bright glowing skin. Herbal teas, such as alfalfa, have been used as a replacement for chocolate, cocoa, and greasy foods for a marked difference in the beauty of the complexion.

To assist in the transportation of oxygen to the brain cells, the body needs a proper supply of potassium for the glands. The kidneys rely upon this supply from the glands to expose fatigue-causing ingredients. The presence of potassium also encourages invigoration and contractions in the kidneys.

Apple cider vinegar is rich in this mineral which helps maintain a hormonal balance in the bloodstream. It may be this source of potassium that assures the healthy and long lives of the people of Vermont who consume a good deal of apple cider vinegar.

Raw or juiced carrots are recommended for the diet to add natural color to the cheeks. Oil of quince, oil of avocado, oil of apricot (kernel), almond oil, sesame oil, what-germ oil, lecithin, lanolin, honey, and natural menthol are all effective natural oils for beauty care.

A beauty formula for the complexion used by the famous Ninon de l'Enclos consisted of boiled fresh milk, lemon juice, and brandy. It was used while still warm as an application for the face.

Wrinkles are creases or furrows in the skin which are created by changes in the deeper skin layers. In youth, the skin has elasticity to overcome such changes but with maturity, the skin loses some of its elastic powers of recoverability.

There are several natural ways of "feeding" the skin which help tone the cells and tissues and in turn, help smooth out some of the wrinkles.

One of the natural treatments for taking care of wrinkled skin is warm olive oil which can be massaged into the forehead. This will replenish lost oils in the various skin layers and has a smoothing effect upon surface wrinkles.

When a few drops of the oil of balm of Gilead is added to barley water, the solution can then be smoothed into the facial tissues to moisturize the skin and help ease wrinkles.

Fresh papaya gives the face a pick-up. Coat the face with mashed papaya for ten minutes while resting in a prone position with the feet elevated by pillows a little higher than the head. After experiencing this complete relaxation, wash the face with warm water and finish by splashing the face with cold water. There is an enzyme in papaya which helps to remove the deadened outer layers of skin and leave you feeling refreshed and rejuvenated.

One of the ancient remedies for wrinkled skin was made by combining the tincture of benzoin, glycerine, honey and, often, a few drops of perfume for scent. Glycerine, rosewater, witch hazel, and honey was another of the ancient concoctions sometimes employed. Honey and glycerine are two of the oldest moisturizers known among the beauty secrets. They are even found in many of the hand lotions of today.

Comfrey is another herb which has been used as a moisturizer for the skin. It contains allantoin which has proven to be an effective moisturizing agent.

Ordinary apple cider vinegar can once again be used in our list of natural applications for beauty. The potassium content works as an antiseptic to cleanse the age-forming debris from the pores and to help tone up the cells and tissues.

Egg on Your Face

This egg facial uplift will help to smooth out wrinkles and revitalize and replenish the cells and tissues of the skin because of its rich, natural cholesterol content. Beat a raw egg with lemon juice and apply to the face and neck. Relax for thirty minutes while you allow the facial to go to work. Wash the mask off with cold water and feel the fresh tingle of your skin.

All of the aforementioned treatments require perseverance along with a good diet for best results to be achieved, so look to your overall care when you think of beauty care.

Eye Sparkle with Beauty

The eyes are never to be overlooked in a discussion of beauty. There is nothing more attractive than vibrant, sparkling eyes; they are a primary vehicle of communication. What can be more exciting than to see the life and beauty of a person in their eyes when you are talking to them? Eyes that are healthy and bright can say yes or no or even maybe; they have an entire language of their own which should not be undermined by an unhealthy and dulled condition.

Sufficient sleep is the first essential in eye beauty and proper diet is the second.

The eyes need their rest to prevent those dark circles and little crow's feet of tension. Sleep is the rejuvenator of our system. Sleep is the favor that you return to your eyes for all of the wonders they give to you.

When considering eye beauty, the importance of proper nutrition can never be overemphasized. Vision is even affected by what we eat and by how we use our eyes. The blood must be healthy with nutritional value in order to properly "feed" the eyes. Undernourished eyes tire quickly and their clarity of vision lessens. Just resting the eyes may not always be sufficient for their revival.

The noted nutritionist, Adelle Davis, has mentioned the importance of nutrition for healthy eyesight. She has reported that many people's vision has actually improved with proper diet. However, good nutrition alone cannot replace the need for eyeglasses.

A vitamin deficiency is usually present when one notices sensitivity to bright lights, or twilight and night blindness.

There are several foods which can be added to the diet which are beneficial for the eyes. Some of these beneficial "eye foods" are blueberries, tomatoes, avocados, eggplant, and sunflower seeds.

As we mentioned in another chapter, the Indians were aware of the need for special eye care in order to assure healthy eyes and improved vision. They were fond of herbal eyewashes. There are a number of additional methods of this sort which have been handed down as folk remedies for eye ease and eye distress.

When the beauty of the eyes has diminished due to overexposure to snow, water, or sun, a natural folk remedy for an eye poultice can be used to relieve burning, reduce inflammation, and restore natural beauty. Folk healers take the white of an egg, beat it slightly, and then spread it on a cloth to be used as a bandage for the eyes. This poultice should be left on the eyes overnight if possible.

Water as an eyewash is invaluable because a majority of the eyefluids and eye tissues are water. Hot and/or cold water applications have a stimulating effect upon the circulation of the eyes. Using the contrasting temperatures, the water will first expand the tissue and fluid content and then it will work on the blood lymph and interstitial fluids or the fluid that exists between the cells. This pumping action of the hot/cold applications helps to improve congestion as well.

The eye is a muscle, and therefore exercise is as important to the eyes as it is to the rest of the body. Eye exercises are usually uncomplicated and can be performed several times a day whenever pressures or daily strain become too great. There are several simple eye exercises that are recommended among the folk healers and yogis of the East.

When exercising the eyes, it is important to sit comfortably in a position which is most relaxing to the rest of the body. Nothing else should be "working" in the body except the eye muscles.

The exercises should be done slowly and quietly without straining or tensing-up the face. When you start moving the eyes in the exercise patterns, try to actually "see" what passes before them and not just go through rapid, unfocused motions.

First, move the eyes upwards, looking as far up as possible without moving the head or wrinkling the forehead. Then, slowly move the eyes downward until you see the cheeks of the face in the same relaxed manner. Do this up-down action completely and quietly for at least four times in each direction.

Secondly, move the eyes sideways as far to the right as possible and then, as far to the left as possible. Following the outer walls of the room, from one ear to the other without moving the head, may help to concentrate your focus and prevent you from "missing" a spot or hurrying. Do four complete cycles.

The third movement is from the upper right hand corner, or eyebrow, to the lower left hand corner, or cheek. Do this up and down action completely four times and then go from the left top corner to the right bottom one in the same way.

The fourth step is to slowly move the eyes in a wide circle following the outlines of your own face if possible, such as the cheeks, side of the eyes, and the eyebrows, four times in one direction and then four times in the opposite. Once again remember to take your time and try to be aware of the relaxation in the rest of the body such as the forehead, shoulders, stomach, and leg muscles. A general feeling of quietness should surround and go through you as you relax. There should be no feeling of rushing, to obtain best results.

Now hold one finger at eye level where you can fully focus upon it and also select one spot far away such as a door knob or cupboard handle that you can also focus upon. The faraway spot should be directly in line with your finger so that you do not need to move your head or your finger in order to see it.

Now look at your finger just long enough for it to come into focus then quickly look away to the faraway spot you have selected until it is completely in focus, then back again at your finger. Do not become fixed upon either point of focus but try to be aware of what you are looking for in order to really *see* your finger and the spot and not just go through the motions with your mind wandering and your body tense. This action should be repeated four complete cycles.

This eye stretch is not only good for the eye

muscles but also for the facial tissues surrounding them.

Squeeze the eyes tightly closed and hold them tight for a slow count of ten. Now open them as wide as possible and hold your focus in a fixed stare for another slow count of ten. Repeat this process for a number of times.

Vigorously rub the palms of your hands together until they produce heat and electricity from the friction. Cup them slightly and place over your open eyes so that no light enters. This action is believed to cause a self-generating electrolyte reaction which supercharges the eyes with natural vitality. This particular "exercise" can be performed any time during the day when a feeling of stress and fatigue overtakes the eyes.

Blinking the eyes during the activities of the day is said to be important for relaxing the eyes. The action of blinking also lubricates and washes the eyes with the tear fluid.

Many naturalists have observed the way that cats rub their eyes with the back of their paws. They believe that gently rubbing the eyes with the knuckles in a similar way can be a relaxing routine for the eyes.

Never stare at objects, instead always keep the eyes moving slightly or scanning the environment. The eyelids should blink rather than be fixed. This will help induce relaxation of the eye muscles which is a key to better vision.

Blinking the eyes under the water has also been found to be beneficial for removing mucus from the eyes and dirt and dust from the lids and lashes.

Some folk healers believe that an exercise of applying compression to the forehead helps to relieve pressure that may be causing tired eyes.

This exercise is done by lying on a bed and lacing the fingers together. The palms are then placed on the forehead. Let the elbows relax fully back onto the bed; the laced fingers should keep the hands together effortlessly. Let the full weight of the hands gently pull the skin toward the eyes. Maintain this position of compression for about fifteen minutes or until sight tension feels as if it is easing away.

The combination of these exercises and herbal preparations for the eyes and rest and good diet should all be considered as being important when seeking a natural beauty way.

Freckles are irregular collections of pigment in the skin which are formed by the pigment cells in an effort to shield the tissues beneath from the sun's rays. They are not merely ugly and unwanted stains on the outside of the skin. People who tan instead of freckling have an even distribution of these pigment-forming cells.

Freckles are also thought to be a sign that the adrenals are large and poorly nourished. Some believe that freckles may tend to disappear when these glands are properly nourished.

There have been various commercial freckle creams on the modern markets but some have proved to be harmful and even dangerous when applied in large doses to the skin.

Many commercial creams which are employed for the removal of freckles depend upon a strong poison, bichloride of mercury, or ammoniated mercury for their success. It is possible for this mercury to be absorbed into the skin and cause a poisoning which could even damage the kidneys. Freckles are situated deep within the skin layers so that any corrosive applications such as mercury, which are strong enough to remove these spots, may also be strong enough to injure the surrounding skin.

Many commercial freckle removers contain salicylic acid as well, which can create a bad rash when applied to the skin or cause the skin to peel. Folk remedies are a much safer source of freckle lightening in the opinion of some naturalists because these harmful ingredients are absent in their formulas.

Lemon juice is a common ingredient in all home remedies where you find the word "lightener." It has also been used to splash over freckles to help lighten their appearance.

A mixture of benzoic acid, tincture of benzoin, rose water and alcohol has been used to fade freckles away.

A lotion can be prepared by combining zinc sulphocarbolate, glycerine, alcohol, orangeflower water and rose water as a folk remedy for freckles. It should be applied after washing and drying the skin.

Fresh elder flowers have been used to remove freckles. The flowers are first covered with water, preferably rain water, distilled water, or water which has been boiled for one hour and cooled. The flowers should be allowed to soak overnight and then strained. The solution may then be used to bathe the freckles twice daily.

Chickweed is another herb that has been used to treat freckles. It must first be mashed in soft water before it is ready for use.

Another wash for freckles or for skin blemishes can be made by placing a cup of centaury herb into two quarts of water with a small amount of castile soap.

There was an old Parisian remedy for skin problems which was made by mixing an ounce of powdered alum with the same amount of lemon juice in a pint of rose water. This concoction should be bottled and then shaken each time before using.

Blackheads are formed when dried, hard, oily materials collect in the oil glands. A dermatologist or physician who specializes in skin problems should always be sought out for any chronic skin ailments. Imbedded dirt must be removed gently or the skin may be easily scarred or disfigured. There are some natural remedies which dissolve and ease blackhead and acne problems besides the ones mentioned above.

There is a home remedy which will nourish the skin and cause an astringent action which is necessary to heal pimples. Lanolin, castor oil, and glycerine are melted together over a mild heat. After the blend has cooled, it can be put into a container and used as an application for pimples.

The natural fatty content is what is of value for the healing process.

Sulphur creates a natural face peel which has been used for acne conditions. Only fresh *Lotio Alba,* or white lotion, should be purchased from a druggist for this purpose. If not more than two weeks old, this rich source of sulphur is effective as a face peel at night after washing with tincture of green soap. It helps to discard dead and infectious skin cells.

Generations of beauty-seekers have used oatmeal for the face to help wash away blackheads. A paste is made of oatmeal, almond meal, orris root, powdered castile soap, and a small amount of hot water. It is gently rubbed into the blackhead area and then left on for an hour to dry. Cold water is then used to rinse the mask away. This will help wash out imbedded dirt if repeated regularly.

The rich vitamin, mineral, and enzyme content of some fruits and vegetables is said to create an astringent and soothing effect on the skin when used for facial preparations to alleviate pimples and blackheads.

The juice from a freshly squeezed cucumber will help heal infections on the face because of its rich vitamin and mineral contents. Tomatoes have been used to treat blotchy and affected skin areas of the face. The raw slices may be applied directly or a mash of the tomato pulp can be used.

A poultice of boiled fresh green beans that have been mashed may be applied to skin blemishes.

After the bean mask has dried, cool water should be used for the rinse.

Cod liver oil has a healing effect if applied liberally to the skin and left as long as possible before washing off in cool water. It is beneficial for the treatment of acne, freckles, blotches, pimples, rashes, cold sores, sunburn, and other skin problems.

Pores become enlarged and dilated when oil glands become blocked and the secretion cannot get out. This causes a hardening of the oily material in the pores. Ice cubes and cold water can be helpful for this condition.

Buttermilk is rich in calcium and phosphorus which helps reduce overly large skin pores and to sterilize the skin. Cotton pads can be used to pat it on the face. After fifteen minutes, it should be rinsed off with cool water.

For those who are suffering from oily skin, lettuce juice can be used daily to combat this condition. The vitamins in the lettuce leaves exert an absorptive action on the excess oil and help drain the film off the skin.

For those whose hands chap easily from constant contact with water, a good hand lotion is made by combining a small amount of benzoin with glycerine. Refined linseed oil can also be combined with rose water and tincture of benzoin for the same purpose.

A natural healing secret from the pioneer days was to use common table salt as a preventive for chapped hands. It is first dampened and rubbed into the hands and then rinsed with cool water. This is also a good way to rid the hands of the unpleasant odors of garlic and onion after cooking.

Glycerine, rosewater, and witch hazel is another combination to provide an effective hand lotion for the relief of chapping.

In a more extreme case of dryness which is accompanied by itching of the skin, slices of raw potato can be rubbed into the area of discomfort. A poultice can also be made from grated potato which has a healing and soothing effect on the affected area.

When confronted with dry facial skin, a mask can be made from the pulp of a ripe avocado. The unsaturated fatty acids found in this beauty source will stimulate the sluggish skin cells and encourage them to produce a healthy supply of sebum, the natural lubricating oil of the skin.

Brittle nails may be the result of a lack of calcium in the system. Besides increasing the amount of calcium-bearing foods in the diet, the nails can be treated directly. Soaking the fingernails in glycerine will help to alleviate this unsightly condition.

For those who aren't worried about freckles but who love to seek out the sun and help insure more even tanning, try reinforcing the blood by eating iron-rich food and drinking iron-rich herb teas before sunbathing.

Excessive sun exposure can cause wrinkles as it tends to dry out the natural moisture of the skin. For this reason one should always keep the skin well lubricated in order to prolong a youthful look.

Baby oil is one method of skin lubrication and also a way to acquire a base tan slowly. For those first exposures to the sun each year, a mixture of baby oil and a sun screen product has been recommended. Once the smooth base tan has been acquired in this way, the continued use of just the baby oil alone will help deepen and enrich the tan while it also helps to lubricate the skin tissues. Continued applications of the oil after your sunbath is helpful to prevent moisture loss. The natural emollient ingredients in baby oil discourage peeling and flaking when used this way and will also help to prevent dry itchy skin.

After showering, a gentle oil rubdown is another aid for smooth, tanned skin. The oil can also be added to your bath water to help keep the skin soft.

Skin that has been exposed to the sun is tender and requires gentle cleansing. Pure baby soap is one way of cleansing tanned skin. Create a lather with the fingertips and gently rub it onto the skin. Baby oil discourages peeling and flaking and will also help to prevent dry itchy skin.

In the case of sunburn, the skin should never be left unattended. A physician should even be consulted in more pronounced cases of sunburn as this may lead to pneumonia or in severe cases, shock. Sunburn should not be taken lightly for the body's reactions should always be treated with respect and care.

For mild cases of sunburn, a solution of glycerine, witch hazel, and sunflower seed oil may prove helpful.

A weak solution of apple cider vinegar is another "old-time remedy" which was probably known to your grandmother even if she wasn't a sun-worshiper herself. The solution can be dabbed onto the sunburned skin generously with saturated cotton pads. If the solution is cool, it will have a more immediate feeling of relief.

Ordinary tea with its tannic acid content can also be used to douse sunburned skin. Whatever method one should choose remember to take the time to care for your skin.

A last note for the sun people, holly thistle as a wash is a good deodorant for the body in the hot weather.

A good bleach for the skin is made by combining lemon, regular peroxide, and witch hazel. One tablespoon of each to one teaspoonful of glycerine should be used.

Another source is cucumber skins rubbed over brown spot areas. Cucumbers are an excellent agent for skin bleaching.

Good grooming and good posture should never be overlooked in beauty culture. Proper nutrition and restful sleep are among the beauty-seeker's best "weapons."

THE SECOND STAGE TO BEAUTY

When discussing beauty and health, the second consideration must be given to the skin. The skin is not usually thought of as a vital organ such as the heart, liver, or lungs although scientists have proven that if the skin fails to function even for a few hours, all of the internal organs can break down.

If the skin were ever coated or completely covered so that no air could possibly penetrate, your body could suffocate.

The millions of pores in the skin are our essential gateway for eliminating waste products from the system. Normally about one quart of moisture is excreted from the millions of sweat glands through the pores in a period of twenty-four hours. The sudorific glands also secrete and discharge a fine oil which lubricates the skin and hair and which also acts as a protective device against invading bacteria.

The excretion of waste products is one of the most important functions of the skin. The skin eliminates more impurities from the body than even the lungs.

Much of the waste material discharged through the skin is in the form of invisible gases called insensible perspiration. Without this vital function of the skin, the blood would retain poisonous waste products and would become more and more toxic and would then be unable to support life. This is why so many herbalists believe that the natural diuretic action of certain herbs is so essential to good health.

Another function of the skin is to regulate the body temperature by preventing the escape of necessary body heat. When the body becomes overheated by exercise, external heat, or fever, the skin performs the opposite task of relieving the tissues by helping the heat to escape.

The skin also functions as an organ of respiration and absorption by the action of taking in oxygen and exhaling poisons and gases.

The skin is also closely connected with all of the great nerve centers as it is an organ of touch and sensation.

The second stage in our stairway to beauty is to be aware of how vital the role of the skin is for our health and for our beauty. The third step is to learn the importance of bathing to assist this function of our skin.

Frequent and proper bathing is essential to remove the impurities that have been deposited upon the skin through perspiration which otherwise would interfere with the further elimination of poisons from the body. The accumulated wastes may even be reabsorbed through the skin and may cause the system to become toxic if they are not bathed away. Unless the skin is free to function as it should, all of the organs of the body will be nourished imperfectly and will be weakened by the impure blood.

Some of the oldest medical authors in history made reference to the benefits of the bath for eliminating disease and encouraging good health. Hippocrates, in his writings, mentions the use of water in various ways as a means of treating disease. Galen was another early advocate of the bath as a natural healing method.

The North American Indians used baths to treat disorders. Among their favorites was the vapor bath.

Mohammed, Charlemagne, and Moses all instructed their people in the use of the bath.

The Romans, Greeks, and Persians have also left records referring to the value of the baths for health. Luxurious establishments were erected for the purpose of the bath during the time of the Roman Empire. It was not until the advent of the Dark Ages that the public baths were abandoned.

In the presence of today's water and air pollution, tension and mental fatigue, the healthful practice of bathing becomes more and more important for our well-being. Certain herbalists maintain that a warm, herbal bath helps to keep harmful bacteria at a minimum besides helping to free the pores by giving a tonic-like refreshment to the body.

The natural fragrance of certain flowers and leaves has a soothing effect upon the mind and feelings. Fragrant lemon grass is still used in the

West Indies, Africa, South America, and the Orient today as a complement to the bath.

It is an old practice in many nations to rub flowers and scented herbs onto their bodies during or after the bath. South Sea Islanders rub the exotic flowers of the Ylang Ylang on the body as part of their toilet.

In India, the leaves of the chaste bush are used to make a warm bath for women after childbirth.

Mugwort was added to the baths of the Roman soldiers to relieve sore and aching muscles.

One of the world's most expensive spices, saffron, was used in Rome by the wealthy ruling classes for the bath. The expense of this herb is due to the fact that three tiny stigmata must be separated from each of 75,000 flowers in order to accumulate one pound of saffron for use.

The American Indians used joe-pye weed, sumach, and witch hazel in addition to other herbs for their remedial baths.

The Haitians placed orange leaves and flowers into the baths of their infants for fragrance.

Herbs have been used in the bath for centuries for a variety of complaints such as nervous insomnia, tension, strain, and sore, aching muscles. The people who have practiced these methods of natural relief have done so because they believe that Nature is still the most welcome healer. They have found that natural healings have caused no side effects, are not narcotic or habit forming, leave no chemical residue in the body's system and that they do not usually lead to adverse reactions either physically or mentally. Natural methods such as herbal baths are more economical than patent medicines and have survived the test of time much longer than many drugs on the market today.

Balm was one of the old herbal bath remedies used to relax muscular tension and ease soreness. Camomile was also added to the bath to ease pains and to relieve body weariness. Mints were frequently employed in baths to comfort the nerves and sinews.

Mugwort was a common remedy for fatigue and muscular aches and pains among the Romans and the Indians. Wild marjoram was a favorite in France and England for the same purpose.

For best results in using herbal baths for muscular aches and pains, soak in the tub for twenty minutes and then massage the muscles preferably with the oil of cajuput or eucalyptus or with camphorated oil. The use of these oils with a massage will help relieve the discomforts even faster because of their deep penetrating action.

Lavender flowers have been used as bath preparations to ease nervousness. In some countries they have even been used to aid in the relief of the pains of rheumatism and gout.

Valerian is another herb valued as a treatment for nervous conditions. One pound of the herb is first boiled for thirty minutes and then the decoction can be added to the bath.

Equal parts of hops and meadowsweet can also be made into a decoction to be poured over the body as a rinse following a bath.

Another decoction of linden flowers or camomile is effective for insomnia when added to the bath. The bath may be followed by linden flower tea to aid in assuring a good night's sleep.

Pine oil bath at the end of the day is another favorite remedy for the relief of tension and strain. It aids in the stimulation of the circulation and to refresh the system.

Sweet flag, or calamus, can be prepared for use in an herbal bath. It is a valuable plant for medicinal purposes in India and was mentioned in the Bible in connection with Moses.

Another ancient healing method from the days of Babylon to relieve tension and stimulate vitality was, after soaking in a warm bath for ten minutes, to rub vigorously with dry salt from the shoulders to the feet. This is said to pick-up the circulation and to melt away tensions even as the salt is dissolving in the water.

To stimulate sluggish skin nerves, mix together finely ground oatmeal, almond meal, finely shaved castile soap, and powdered orris root with the fragrance of violet. Rub the bag over the skin following a tub soak for a new glow.

Cold baths are never recommended for use by the aged or for those suffering from heart trouble, obesity, or neurasthenia.

Hot baths are known to increase the circulation by driving the blood near to the surface of the skin, causing the veins to enlarge. They are also known to create a sense of heaviness in the head leaving the bather feeling fatigued and weak.

Warm baths are the most advisable as they do not shock the body and will always leave the bather feeling refreshed.

A warm bath can be used to help increase the circulation when a person is unable to exercise and has cold hands and feet. The English added a decoction of marigold, nettle, and bladder wrack to the water to aid in this purpose.

The skin is protected by an acid mantle which is destroyed by the use of harsh alkaline soaps. Soap is an irritant to this natural acid base of the skin because of its caustic alkalies and fats which penetrate the skin's protective layer and leach out the protective emulsion from the skin.

This acid mantle of the skin is referred to as its pH factor. Normal skin has a pH factor from four to six. Some tests have indicated that a normal skin with a pH factor of four rises to a pH seven, one minute after the face had been washed with soap. Cider vinegar can be applied to the skin after bathing to maintain the normal pH factor.

The soaps made from the balsam of Peru are a source of soft, creamy lather. Baby soaps and non-detergent soaps such as Ivory are the most gentle on the skin.

The most important function of bathing is to remove the dead cells from the surface of the skin so that the pores are free to operate properly. A natural sponge can be used to scrub the whole body to get this desired effect.

If suffering from dry skin, use soap on the entire

body only once a week. The rest of the time, merely scrub the skin well and soap only the underarms, genitals, and any areas exposed to externals.

If the skin is particularly dry and itchy, there is an old remedy which can still be tried today. Place one pound of oatmeal into a cloth bag, secure, and immerse in your bath water. Soak for twenty minutes while you gently scrub the skin with the oatmeal bag to help the skin feel soft again.

Scrubbing will also increase the circulation and will leave you with a healthy glow.

The records of Babylon, 604-561 B.C., make reference to King Nebuchadnezzar's "lion strength." He had incredible vitality and personally led armies all through the Middle East to victories in battle. The palace scribes of the day attributed his astonishing mental and physical health to the special "washings" which he took once a week.

Historians believe that this ancient health restorative practiced by King Nebuchadnezzar was the forerunner of the Turkish bath. It is still thought to be a beneficial way of cleansing the body of toxic wastes. It provides a self-washing method that purges the glands and internal organs so that they can function without the accumulation of grime, mucus, sludge, and waste.

To practice this cleansing procedure at home, first, drink plenty of fresh water to avoid dehydration because the Turkish bath produces perspiration in order to cast off wastes. Keep the bathroom door closed throughout the bath. Fill the tub with comfortable hot water (105 degrees and up). Sit outside the tub and allow the temperature to open the pores by inducing perspiration. After thoroughly perspiring, rub your body with a rough cloth in order to remove the mucus perspiration from the skin's surface.

If the tub water is comfortably hot, relax into the bath at this point and remain in the water for ten minutes.

Stand in the tub and allow the water to run out of the tub. Turn on the shower or use a faucet hose to rinse in cool water and close the pores.

Dry off completely and lie down in a room that is comfortably warm (70-80 degrees) and feel the effects of your Turkish bath.

This self-inducement of natural perspiration helps to rid the body of accumulated wastes and infectious toxic mucus-sludge that could otherwise possibly cause distress in the body. This also helps normalize the body temperature, build resistance to colds, relaxes the nervous system, and replenishes the bloodstream. Perhaps Nebuchadnezzar knew what he was doing after all.

Man throughout the ages has always acquired aromatic pleasure from the perfumes of flowers, herbs, and the gums of tropical trees. Records which date back to Nebuchadnezzar in 570 B.C., King Tut, and the Arabian Nights all make reference to the use of aromatic plants.

There are a number of combinations of herbs for perfuming the bath. Any aromatic botanical such as rosemary may be substituted in this concoction for a fragrant bath experience. Mix ten parts of borax crystals with four parts of cut, not powdered, orris roots, four parts of khus-khus roots, four parts of rose leaves, and one part each of benzoin, sandalwood, and rose geranium.

An assortment of herbs such as calamus, bay, rosemary, camomile, and marigold flowers may be added to boiling water, covered, and simmered for ten or fifteen minutes. Strain and use as another bath fragrance or as a warm rinse after the bath.

Roses. The rose has been associated with goddesses since ancient times. The preparation of *attar of roses* is derived from an East Indian legend. A sultana of Jehanghir was said to have filled the bath of the palace garden with rose water. The action of the sun soon caused the oil particles to become concentrated and to float to the surface. An attendant thought the water had become polluted, so the legend goes, and began to skim off the floating particles. The globules then began to burst and expel the perfume preparation.

Sandalwood. Sandalwood is a popular incense introduced by the religious ceremonies of the Chinese and East Indians. It is also mixed with rice paste to make scented candles in China. King Solomon's temple was supposed to have been made of sandalwood.

Lavender. The deep fragrant aroma of lavender was a favorite in the Roman bath. Its name is derived from the Latin word which means "to wash." The flowers can also be dried and used as a sachet and moth repellent. One old folk remedy was to mix the flowers of the lavender with cinnamon, nutmeg, and cloves into a powder and serve as a drink for "panting and passion of the heart."

Khus-Khus. This favorite of the West Indies is found in almost every market place on each of the islands. The dried roots are used as a delicate sachet and also to repel insects.

Lovage. This plant has a small, yellow flower and is grown for its fragrant bouquet. The flower was associated with folklore as an additive for the bath to increase one's ability to be loved. The seeds of lovage were used formerly in a medicinal preparation for "falling sickness." The juices have been used in "witches ointment." The roots can be kept for many years to use for their fragrance.

With the hard water in which most of us bathe and the polluted air to which we are exposed, an oil or water softener should always be used in the bath to aid in moisturizing the skin.

A good natural bath oil can be prepared by mixing one pint of vegetable oil with a small amount of liquid shampoo.

A bag of meadowsweet placed in the bath water is a good beauty preparation.

Peppermint leaves can be heated to boiling, then simmered for five minutes and strained. When this decoction is added to cider vinegar, it is a soothing solution for the bath.

Rosemary, lavender, and comfrey placed in a muslin bag make for a refreshing hot water bath.

Camomile and nettle tea are fine beauty teas to be used externally and internally. Yarrow tea has also been mentioned as a wash to achieve velvet-like skin.

Hyssop is a cleanser and beautifier when prepared as an infusion and used as a wash. It is a native plant of Asia and Europe. The aromatic oil extracted from the green parts of hyssop are used to make English eau de cologne.

A "milk bath" preparation can be made by combining five parts of oatmeal with one part each of almond meal and orris root, and one-half part of castile soap. This assemblage can then be added to the bath in bags for a milky, fragrant cleanser and beautifier for the skin.

Lavender flowers, rosemary leaves, dried mint, comfrey roots, and thyme can be mixed together loosely in a muslin bag, steeped in boiling water, then added to a warm bath as another "beauty formula." It was popular with the French beauty, Ninon de l'Enclos, who was known for her youthful appearance even at the age of seventy. If there is any connection between her use of the herbal bath and her radiant appearance, one would tend to assume that habitual use was a factor.

Helen of Troy's Beauty Bath

This herbal-vinegar bath is said to be the legendary beauty secret of Helen of Troy. Rosemary, lavender, rue, and camphor are first soaked in white wine vinegar for a few hours. After straining, the liquid can be added to warm bath water for legendary Grecian beauty.

HERBS AND THE FEET

When considering cleanliness as a necessity for good health, the feet must not be forgotten as an important part of the body which need special care. Few people take time to care for or even notice their feet today. Feet are seldom allowed to be bare to breathe; their arches are strained into unnatural positions in the high-heeled fashion shoes of the day. They are subjected to blisters, bunions, calluses, and cramps. They get bumped, scuffed, pinched, and over-heated in the course of an average day. Our feet should not only be treated more kindly because of the service they do for us but for hygienic purposes as well.

Waste materials and poisons from the body continually collect on the bottoms of the feet and form a coating over the pores. The feet must be washed thoroughly and regularly for this reason to prevent the accumulation of rejected poisons from being reabsorbed into the body.

There are a number of herbal foot baths that have been passed down through history which have been used for treating tired and diseased feet. Several are mentioned by Father Kneipp in his writings, *My Water Cure*. Herbal foot baths have been recommended to dissolve the accumulation on the bottoms of the feet, cleanse the pores, and also for the treatment of feet suffering from sweating, athlete's foot, corns, ingrown toe nails, calluses, and bunions.

All of the parts of hay can be used for sanitary foot bath by pouring boiling water over the assortment, covering, and letting the mixture stand until it is cool enough for the feet. This decoction has also been advised for use in conjunction with warm and cold foot baths, alternating to first one and then the other; ten minutes in the warm and then one minute in the cold for a period of about half an hour. This procedure should always end in the cold bath.

To absorb excessive perspiration, a powder is made by some folk healers to rub onto the feet or to shake into the shoes. Powdered orris root is simply mixed with zinc oxide and ordinary talcum.

Another folk remedy for perspiring feet and offensive foot odor is made by combining vinegar, alcohol, and cologne water. This solution can be sponged onto the feet every night for a week.

Corns and Calluses

Calluses often result because of the toes' effort to protect themselves from irritation. Result: shoe pressure will cause a knotty thickening of the skin. A hard core forms in the center of this knotty protrusion, which in turn presses onto the nerves that are beneath the skin and causes pain.

For the relief of corns and calluses, the feet should be soaked in hot water at bedtime. A small piece of lemon peel should then be bound over the corn or callus with the pulpy side towards the foot. This should not be removed until morning and the whole procedure should be repeated at bedtime for the next four or five days.

Another foot bath for corns, calluses, and bunions is made by adding a cup of yarrow leaves and a tablespoon of salt to three quarts of hot water.

Castor oil is used by some herbalists to rub into corns and calluses as a softener.

Olive oil is used as a lubricant for corns and dry skin. It has also been used as an application to the toe nails to prevent brittleness or splitting.

Gum arabic mucilage is another application to soften corns or calluses.

After soaking the feet in hot water, lemon juice or kerosene may be applied nightly to treat corns.

Sliced onion which has been soaked in vinegar for twenty-four hours can be bandaged to the corn to be left on overnight.

Bunions

A bunion occurs when the joint at the base of the big toe becomes inflamed. Improperly styled shoes which crowd the big toe and cause too much pressure on the joint are usually the cause of bunions.

A bunion pad is thought to bring relief as it is designed to give the painful inflammation of the joint a chance to subside.

A daily hard-pressure massage directly on the bunion swelling will help break up the bunion-forming deposits at the joint.

Athlete's Foot

The presence of athlete's foot can be detected by reddish eruptions on the feet. These are followed by a cracking of the skin between the toes and a watery discharge, which is accompanied by itching at all stages. It is a highly infectious condition which is caused by a fungus and can be contracted by walking barefoot, particularly on moist floors such as bathrooms and swimming pools.

The blossoms of red clover are boiled until thick to be used as a direct herbal application to the affected areas.

Apple cider vinegar, either plain or diluted, is another natural remedy in the relief of that foot discomfort.

MORE ABOUT
WATER AND DISEASE

Hippocrates, in 500 B.C., wrote about the use of water to be taken internally and to be applied externally to combat diseases. The Persians, Greeks, and Romans all erected monumental public buildings for bathing. During the times of epidemics and pestilences, these baths were considered the safest refuge from the devastations of infectious diseases.

Two thousand years ago, the Latin physicians, Celus and Galen, considered bathing invaluable. Galen believed that proper bathing combined with the application of friction to the body should be regarded as medicinal. Methods of bathing were later used to combat fevers, infections, and internal disorders.

Public vapor baths became popular in the Europe of the 1600's. The self-cleansing action of the steam helped to scrub out the impurities of the insides, wash the mucus-covered system, and restore good health to ailing patients.

The notability of water healing became more evident at the beginning of the next century. *Cu-*

riosities of Common Water, a health book published in 1723, cited water as an inexpensive and simple remedy for many ills.

In the 1850's, a German water healer, Victor Priesnitz, came onto the scene and gained a reputation for an ability to use water to cure many patients abandoned by the medical profession of the day as incurable.

The Americans soon heard of the "new" water cures only to learn that the Indians had been practicing the art of natural water healing for many generations. The Indians even used contrast baths to ease stiffness and swollen joints.

As with all of the natural remedies, none can be effective if used to the exclusion of other healthful practices such as a proper diet of simple and natural foods, sufficient rest, exercise, fresh air, and controlled sunlight exposure.

Father Sebastian Kneipp, who became known for curing the Bright's disease in Archduke Joseph of Austria (1892), reported the failures of water healing if the patient continued to abuse his body by overwork, poor food, and a lack of exercise and then looked to water healing as the sole answer to his problem.

The Swiss and mountain healers of that land have long realized that nature's mineral-rich waters are important for a healthy blood stream which they consider our river of life.

Water is a nutrient, second only to oxygen in health benefit, and it helps regulate the body's processes and temperature. About ninety percent of blood plasma is water.

The average person should drink at least six to eight glasses of water daily. Two glasses should be consumed an hour before each meal, for it is vital to the function of intestinal regularity.

After consumption, water can be absorbed into the blood stream to help purify the body by cleansing it of poisons and waste matter. This purifying action can be noted by increased waste secretions and increased perspiration.

Water aids in the washing and rebuilding of the tissue cells and all body fluids. It helps to activate the skin function and, as a result, increases circulation. This in turn helps to build resistance to colds and allergic tendencies.

Chlorinated water, because of the chlorine itself, destroys the vitamin E content in the body. Spring water, mineral water, or boiled chlorinated water is more advisable as a source of good health.

External water treatment has been used to correct conditions of clogged arteries, digestive disturbances, stiff, aching and swollen joints, nerve distress, glandular irregularity, internal organ disorder, allergic tendencies, loss of vitality and premature aging, as well as a lack of energy. When proper water healing is used in combination with healthful diet, rest, and exercise it is a beneficial method of treatment.

In a report of a case of high cholesterol count with the existing possibility of developing into arteriosclerosis and other conditions of arthritis, a self-washing program was recommended. The suggested proposal consisted of a fifteen minute hot shower followed by a cold shower. During the cold shower, the patient was instructed to hop around and rub his hands over his body and after a few moments, to step out and dry thoroughly. The hot shower opened the pores and the steam created an artery-scrubbing sensation.

The benefits of a hot-cold water program such as this are in the reaction of the circulatory system. The steam dilates the blood vessels of the skin, allowing a fresh supply of blood to rush to the surface. The blood then rushes through the body in an effort to cool off the system.

The cold water then works as a contrasting action to constrict the blood vessels. This then produces a quick flushing of the fats, cholesterol, and wastes through the liver and kidneys to cause rapid elimination.

In this way it is thought that this self-washing technique will dilate, constrict, and flush cholesterol from the body, thus burning it by elevation of temperature.

This program, once again, can only be fully effective if used in conjunction with a cleansing, nutritious diet, healthy exercise, and sufficient, restful sleep.

If you have trouble "getting started" in the mornings, this program may be of special interest to you. This method of bathing will not only stimulate the circulation and increase vitality, but will help build up a resistance to winter cold, lower the blood pressure, and enhance the skin.

The first procedure is to relax for a full fifteen minutes in a hot tub of water, 104 to 112 degrees.

Next, release the tub drain and stand up. Start the shower with lukewarm water and gradually decrease the temperature, turning as you do so that all of the body benefits from the shower stream.

The aftereffects of the hot tub will keep your warm blood pumping through the body so that you will not actually feel cold as the temperature changes. As the water gets colder, rub the body vigorously where the shower stream is striking and if you begin to feel cold, stop the shower immediately and step into a large dry towel and rub with gusto.

There are other benefits of hot and cold baths for the body and they were not unknown to our ancestors. The use of cold water to revive someone from a faint is still a common practice of stimulation today. Hydrotherapy has developed into a method of natural healing from practices just as simple as this.

There are many nerve endings on the surface of the body. Some act as receivers for heat and some are receivers of cold. The use of contrast temperature bathing is to help revive sluggish nerves.

Hot water works as a relaxer to smooth out tense muscle cells where they are bunched together. The heat slows the flow of the blood because the constant temperature does not allow for a variance in the amount of circulating blood. This causes an increase in the amount of blood in the surface of the body and creates a feeling of comforting warmth and relaxation.

In a case of "goose bumps" of the skin when the

small blood vessels become constricted and the muscular and elastic tissues in and under the skin contract, cold water can cause a sensation of stimulation and can revitalize the circulation. Cold water will cause an immediate dilation of the constricted blood vessels and a rush of blood will warm the skin and give it a pink glow.

When suffering from very cold extremities such as minor frost bite, an old folk remedy was to first soak the cold hands or feet for a few minutes in comfortably hot water, then to briefly plunge them into cold water, then back into warm water and so on for a dozen times, always ending in warm water. This method slowly warms those afflicted areas by stimulating the circulation.

A modern natural healer, Dr. Louis Savas, has recommended cold packs for severe muscular tension in the shoulders and at the base of the neck. He suggests wringing out a small wet towel, folding and placing it in the freezer to freeze. For temporary relief of muscular discomfort, apply the frozen cloth as a compress to the shoulder area. This action will cause the blood to rush to the area to warm and relax the tense muscles.

For muscular stiffness around the spinal area, a hot shower has been prescribed by some naturalists for simple and temporary relief. Stand with the back to the water with the feet comfortably apart. Bend the knees slightly and support the weight of the body with the hands on the knees. Feel the hot spray on the back and gently arch first the lower back, then the upper. Raise first one hip and then the other in a rolling fashion. In this manner you gently allow the water to massage the moving muscles of the back and help to relieve muscular congestion. The movement is similar to the stretching and arching of a cat that is naturally aware of self-massage and spine-rolling for relaxing.

A tub of shallow hot water can also be used to soothe a stiff back. Lie on the back in about four inches of comfortably hot water with the bottoms of the feet flat against the wall at the foot of the tub. Slowly inch your way toward the feet, allowing the knees to become more and more bent and the spine to become flatter and more completely covered by the hot water. If this position is comfortable, the hips can be rolled gently so that the muscles are moving and stretching and gradually expanding in the warmth of the water.

Oxygen is the elixir of life for the blood and all of the body cells. It passes into the bloodstream through seven hundred fifty million air sacs or cells. One quarter of the body's blood passes over the lungs each second in order to leave off the carbon dioxide gas and pick up that life force, oxygen, to carry back to the cells.

An oxygen bath has been used as an old folk remedy to aerate the bloodstream by helping to restore the oxygen that has been depleted from the system. This method is ideal for those suffering from exhaustion, tiredness, and the shortness of breath resulting from respiratory difficulties.

To self-oxygenate in twenty minutes, add sodium perborate, manganese borate, and ordinary baking soda to your bath water. The results of soaking in this bubbly, oxygen bath, which is not unlike bathing in champagne except for its economical advantage, are extremely stimulating and revitalizing.

Water to Combat Insomnia

This method of self-inducing sleep is as old as time but still is considered valuable by some naturalists. Soaking in a warm tub will generally bring on a feeling of over-all relaxation. The action of the heat will numb the delicate nerve endings of the skin and soothe the muscular condition. To encourage sleep, following the warm soak, you merely pat the body dry. Vigorous rubbing will tend to stimulate the nerve ends again and to revive the body rather than to relax it for sleep.

Foot Bath for Sleep

The hot foot bath is another natural sleep-relaxant. Soaking the feet for fifteen minutes in a hot foot bath will improve the circulation by sending blood rushing through the blood vessels of the body. This is beneficial for relieving tension, restoring normal circulation and inducing a feeling of relaxation.

Cool water should be poured onto the feet as a finish and then they should be dried thoroughly and gently. Alcohol or cider vinegar may then be used to massage the feet, ankles, and calves in an upward motion. If the feet and legs are suffering from dryness, olive oil or castor oil may be used for the same purpose.

HAIR IS BEAUTY

As in the case of facial and skin beauty, for lustrous, healthy hair a balanced diet must be maintained. Any disease or illness which infects the body or retards vitality directly affects the condition of the hair.

The source of beautiful hair is a pure bloodstream, nourished with essential foods. The daily diet should be rich in protein foods such as nuts, beans, peas, cheese, eggs, fish, and meat. The bloodstream carries nutrients to the scalp so that vital blood enriching minerals should also be obtained by eating plenty of fresh raw fruits and vegetables. The vitamins necessary for stimulating the growth factors are also found in fresh fruits and vegetables.

The intake of enzymes, which help transform nutrients into the ingredients which help to grow hair, is also essential for the healthy hair diet.

The contents of your diet will actually affect the shine and elasticity of your hair, so reconsider your diet when seeking hair beauty.

Loss of hair is often brought about by nervous diseases, sinusitis, worry, fear, mental disorders, skin diseases, or excessive shampooing and harsh unnatural brushes.

Iron deficiency can encourage the loss of hair while riboflavin is a necessary element for the stimulation of the normal hair growth which is one inch every six weeks.

Sulphur in the diet is important for luxuriant hair. Mullein, eyebright, and stinging nettle are all sulphur containing herbs. Sulphur vegetables should always be eaten raw and never boiled.

Zinc-containing wheat germ is a valuable asset for the growth of healthy hair.

Inositol is a salicylic sugar which plays a part in fat metabolism. In the presence of total inositol deficiency, you could become completely hairless. Brewer's yeast, wheat germ, carrots, apples, bananas, molasses, tomatoes, strawberries, lettuce, cantaloupe, and dried peas are all good sources of inositol.

Diseased thyroid gland has previously led to the loss of hair. The iodine found in seafood, seaweed, and sarsaparilla is essential for a healthy thyroid condition.

The use of permanent-wave solution has been a cause of loss of hair in some instances. Hair dye and hair bleaches have caused clumps of hair to break off at the crown.

To stimulate the growth of hair, wheat germ, cod liver oil, and lecithin are all necessary in your diet.

Cider vinegar may be simmered with rosemary leaves, peach leaves, and southernwood ashes to aid in hair growth.

A four day plan for hair regrowth would consist of: On the first day the hair should be parted into small sections and white iodine should be applied to the scalp with a cotton swab.

On the second day after parting the hair into sections, a small amount of castor oil should be massaged into the scalp until it is absorbed.

The third day should be a repeat of the first white iodine application and on the fourth day, the castor oil is again massaged into the scalp. On this day, the addition of a hot towel is used to steam the oil into the scalp after the massage. The steam treatment should be applied four times and then the hair allowed to dry naturally.

Coconut oil is also a source of stimulation for the hair follicles.

Coconut oil can be used regularly as a massage for the scalp to promote hair health. The additional use of steam treatments helps the oil to penetrate deep into the scalp to nourish the roots of the hair.

Coconut oil is beneficial for the hair because of its rich content of phosphorus, potassium, and natural unsaturated fatty acids. These elements all work as lubricants to stimulate the function of the hair shaft and hair follicles.

Premature graying can also be an indication of poor or insufficient nourishment, so once again the diet is important.

Studies have shown that graying of the hair is related to the action of the adrenal glands. It follows then that stress and strain may actually bring about graying.

The lack of certain B vitamins has some effect on hair color. Calcium is also an important factor in maintaining the hair's natural color. Calcium deficiency is usually detected by dull, brittle hair which has a tendency to split and will not hold a set.

There are several herbal concoctions which have darkened graying hair. Their success depends upon the rest of the diet.

Stinging nettle or cider vinegar can be boiled in water as a hair tonic for this purpose.

Sage has been prepared and used in the same way. The longer the sage boils, the darker the color of the rinse will become.

Honey, rosemary leaves, and grape tendrils have been prepared together as an infusion for darkening gray hair.

Sage leaves and green tea have been boiled together as a solution for this purpose as well.

Wind, rain, and sun have a drying effect upon the hair which deadens the natural color. The natural emulsion of oil rubbed into the scalp can help to replenish the natural oil supply that has been lost.

The high unsaturated content of castor oil can help put life back into the hair color. It can be used as a massage for the scalp the night before washing the hair. Steaming the hair with hot towels after applying the oil will help to speed up the process of penetration.

Olive oil can be used in the same way. Massage warm olive oil into the scalp, steam with hot wet towels for extra benefit, then follow with the use of a natural shampoo.

A regular use of these oil treatments helps rejuvenate the hair color by restoring natural oils to the hair.

During the era of the Royalists of Europe, the women used a natural hair dye for beauty. They boiled equal parts of vinegar, lemon juice, and powdered litharge for thirty minutes over a slow fire in a porcelain-lined kettle. The mixture was then combed through the hair as a natural dye.

Some nutritionists have suggested that blackstrap added to the diet will help to recolor hair. It can take from two weeks to one year for this process to be complete. One method was to mix blackstrap, natural honey, and apple cider vinegar in a jar, shake and then add to the daily drinking water. Blackstrap can also be added to coffee, protein drink, and yogurt to obtain the same results.

Blackstrap is known to be rich in B vitamins and minerals such as iron and copper. All of these components are used in the natural recoloring of animal fur.

Shampooing the hair creates a loss of calcium, phosphorus, iron, and nitrogen from the hair, therefore it should be done in moderation. Food rich in these minerals should also be an important part of the diet to help restore these components to the hair.

American women have a reputation for "overwashing" their hair and for all of the money spent in beauty salons, they have the least healthy hair in the world. Italians have the most beautiful hair in the world. It may be due, in part, to the large amount of olive oil consumed by the Italian people.

Olive oil can be substituted for vegetable oil in the daily diet to enhance hair beauty. It can also be used externally for a scalp treatment before shampooing. If this method is used, the oil may also be rubbed into the ends of the hair and left for thirty to sixty minutes before shampooing. This will help to eliminate split ends and will add body to the hair.

Natural Shampoos

Egg shampoo was a popular method of health care several generations ago and can still be used today. The rich silicon and sulphur content of the egg, plus its natural fatty acids, help nourish the hair. There are two preparations for egg shampoo.

The first is to beat an egg yolk with a cup of skim milk until it is of a foam consistency. It then can be rubbed thoroughly into the scalp and rinsed with clear warm water.

The second preparation is to beat two or three raw eggs and then to rub them into your wet hair. After the head has been thoroughly "lathered," rinse with lukewarm water. A teaspoonful of white vinegar in a quart of lukewarm water may then be used as a rinse. Brush the hair thoroughly while it is drying.

An extract of yucca plant roots, *yuccarone,* is a natural ingredient which has been used for centuries by the southwestern American Indians as a shampoo. It can be found commercially today in some salons.

Ordinary pure castile soap is a mild and soothing shampoo for the hair. It will also soothe itching and will promote a favorable scalp condition.

Castile soap is used in a Spanish shampoo. One-half pound is sliced and put into a porcelain pot with two quarts of warm water. As it is boiled, the soap will dissolve. When the solution has cooled it will be of a thin creamy consistency. Add one-quarter pint of ethyl alcohol and let the mixture stand in a warm room for a few days. A small portion can then be used as a natural shampoo. Rinse the head in cool water after use.

When shampooing the hair, water temperature must be an important consideration. Warm water is better for hair than hot water.

Combs and brushes should be washed each time the hair is shampooed. A small amount of ammonia may be added to the wash water to help protect against dandruff and falling hair.

One of the best hair washes and hair rinses known for centuries is made from rosemary. An infusion can be prepared by steeping a small amount in boiling water to use externally. In some countries the infusion is combined with borax and used as a preventive against premature balding. The Mexicans mash rosemary and then steep it in pure alcohol for several days to be used as a treatment for falling hair. The solution is then vigorously rubbed into the scalp twice a day.

Rosemary has also been combined with raspberry leaves and red sage as a preparation to be brushed through the hair for sheen. The herbs are saturated with boiling water, covered, cooled, and strained for use.

Modern shampoos, tonics, and hair conditioners employ the use of the oil of rosemary as a main ingredient. Rosemary oil is also found in cosmetic soaps, perfumes, and eau de cologne.

An oil for the hair can be made by combining the oil and leaves of rosemary with egg yolk, soapwort, papaya leaves, stinging nettle, yarrow, sunflower seed oil, and glycerine.

Because of heavy pollution and modern day tensions, dandruff is not an uncommon ailment with the average American.

There are several herbal remedies that have been used throughout the ages for the treatment of dandruff.

The Indiana Botanic Gardens prepared a formula to be used as a warm hair wash instead of shampoo as a treatment for dandruff. Its contents include haar wurzel, jaborandi leaves, sage leaves, camomile flowers, and peach tree leaves which are to be soaked all together in cider vinegar and water.

The willow tree leaves and bark have been used to rid the hair of dandruff.

When suffering from a scaly scalp, a salt remedy can be tried. A paste is first made by adding five tablespoons of water to a cup of packed salt. It is then rubbed into the scalp and left for five minutes. Brush the hair briskly and then shampoo.

In the case of minor scalp itching, a special

form of liquid soap may be used for a shampoo to help nourish the scalp and ease the itching. Saponified coconut oil can be obtained from a pharmacy for this purpose as it is gentler, more effective and lower in price than most commercial shampoos. It helps reduce dandruff and promotes a general feeling of good health.

Herb Rinses and Tonics

After shampooing, the scalp is left in an alkaline state and should be restored to its normal state of acidity. Lemon or vinegar rinses help recover the natural pH factor to the scalp after shampooing.

The twigs of wild cherry as a hair tonic, and plantain and shepherd's purse to improve hair texture and sheen are also good. Peppergrass, marshmallow leaves, and mullein leaves all nourish and brighten the hair.

Sage and camomile rinses are used in some modern salons.

The leaves and bark of the willow tree can be soaked in a cup of boiled water until tepid. This rich supply of natural minerals can then be used to soak the scalp and to nourish the hair shafts to stimulation.

After shampooing, a small amount of mayonnaise may be left on the hair for one hour to help relieve a dry condition. The natural fatty acids help nourish and feed the hair and promote the flow of oil from the sebaceous glands. This conditioner should then be shampooed lightly and rinsed.

In the case of extremely oily hair, one tablespoon of salt may be dissolved in your wave-set lotion to soak up the excess oil.

To add protein and body to your hair, any vegetable oil such as sesame, peanut, castor, or olive may be used as a wave-set. It can be combined with a small amount of solubilized lanolin such as solubilized isopropyl or acetylated lanolin. This mixture should not be rinsed out of the hair after it has been applied. This will help hold a set for days.

Ordinary tea was used as a rinse for the hair before the days of commercial shampoos. A mild acid tea will leave the hair with a glossy sheen.

A teaspoon of camomile leaves can be steeped in hot water to apply as a hair tonic. Allow it to dry in the hair, then brush and set. It will help bring out a rich, natural color in the hair.

Lemon juice will help bring out a natural glow in the hair and can also be considered a natural, mild bleach. You can also use it for a case of oily hair. Simply sprinkle lemon juice with water onto the hair; allow it to dry; brush and set.

One pound of rosemary can be stewed in a quart of water for five hours and then strained. Add one-half pint of bay rum to this herbal tonic to rub into the roots of the hair twice a day.

Apple cider vinegar is a common treatment for the hair as its potassium content will give the hair shine and body. It should be mixed with water to use as a rinse after shampooing.

If troubled with dry frizzy hair, the hair can be rinsed with wheat germ oil after shampooing. Follow this with a vinegar rinse and your hair will be tame again.

Nettle, pepper, sage, henna leaves, or burdock are each mentioned in folklore herbal care for the hair. Any one of them may be steeped in boiling water for thirty minutes. The solution is then massaged into the scalp, allowed to dry, and then combed or brushed as usual. Each of these herbs is rich in minerals and enzymes which act as stimulants to the hair.

A hair shaft is flat and porous and curls up when it absorbs moisture and becomes shorter. Hair curls when soaked in an alkaline solution and then heated. A hair-curling solution can be made by mixing gum tragacanth, water, glycerine, and rose compound oil. After standing for twenty-four hours, it is then strained and bottled for use.

Another solution for the purpose of curling the hair has been prepared by mixing gum arabic, rosewater, sesame oil, wheat germ oil, lanolin, and glycerine.

Apple pectin has been used for curling also.

Besides using ordinary lemon juice to lighten the hair naturally, camomile flower tea has been used to highlight blond hair.

Blonde-haired women of the past used marigold flowers for tinting their hair.

Head Massage for Health Care

Head massage is recommended to help increase circulation and to stimulate hair growth. It also helps to ease tightness of the scalp which is caused by tension. When the scalp is tight, a sufficient amount of fatty tissue is not allowed beneath the skin of the scalp. Increase of nervous tension is believed to increase the amount of dandruff as well.

To increase circulation among the hair cells, take a deep breath and bend forward from the waist until the head is lower than the shoulders; keep the knees bent.

While holding the breath in this position, use the fingers to gently knead the skin starting from the neck and working up in front of the ears to the scalp.

Release the fingers and gently use your palms to apply pressure to the forehead.

Exhale as you come to a standing position and drop the hands. This should all be done very calmly and casually in a well-ventilated room. The complete sequence should be repeated five consecutive times daily to experience a tremendous flow of oxygenated blood revitalizing the hair and scalp.

The ancients prepared a solution to use with massage to help conditions of dandruff and falling hair. They used a tea made from the leaves and bark of the willow tree.

Nettle, pepper grass, sage, henna leaves, or burdock can also be steeped in boiling water and used as a scalp massage after adding a small amount of boric acid. The hair should be rinsed after the massage first in lukewarm and then in cold water.

An old herbal hair treatment of the Spanish gypsies was to mix one ounce of spirits of rosemary
with one pint of warm water. This was then mixed
into the yolk of one egg with a pinch of borax.
They suggested that this mixture be rubbed into
the scalp for five minutes and then washed and
rinsed.

Get the Brush

Daily and proper hair brushing is essential for
hair vitality and sheen. Plastic and artificial bris-
tles should never be used on the hair as they tend
to tear the hair shafts and irritate the scalp.

Brushing regularly with a natural bristle brush
distributes the oil to the full length of each hair
which helps to make the hair shine. Brushing is
the scalp's exercise. It loosens and removes dry
dead skin, increases circulation, removes lint and
dirt, and helps stimulate each follicle to make it
come alive.

To get the best results from brushing, bend forward from the waist and let the head hang down.
Brush away from the head, from the scalp to the
hair ends in order to let hair breathe and to per-
mit a rush of oxygen-bearing blood to nourish the
follicles.

Use long firm strokes and take the time for that
old "one hundred strokes a day" remedy whenever possible. This is also a more natural and
healthy way to give the hair style and body without harmful "teasing."

After brushing the hair forward over the head, just "flick" the hair back as you stand. The hair will be aerated and you will feel somewhat rejuvenated.

DEFINITION OF MEDICINAL PROPERTIES OF HERBS

ALTERATIVE: Producing a healthful change without perceptible evacuation

ANODYNE: Relieves pain

ANTHELMINTIC: An agent which expels worms

ANTIBILIOUS: Acts on the bile, relieving biliousness

ANTIEMETIC: Stops vomiting

ANTIEPILEPTIC: Relieves fits

ANTIPERIODIC: Arrests morbid periodical movements

ANTHILITIC: Prevents the formation of calculi in the urinary tract

ANTIRHEUMATIC: Relieves rheumatism

ANTISCORBUTIC: Helps prevent scurvy

ANTISEPTIC: Opposed to putrefaction

ANTISPASMODIC: Helps relieve spasms

APERIENT: Gently laxative, without purging

AROMATIC: Causes contraction and arrests discharges

ASTRINGENT: Causes contraction and arrests discharges

CARMINATIVE: Expels air from the bowel

CATHARTIC: Evacuating the bowels

CEPHALIC: Used in ailments of the head

CHOLAGOGUE: Increases the flow of bile

CONDIMENT: Improves flavor of food

DEMULCENT: Soothing, relieves inflammation

DEOBSTRUENT: Removes obstructions

DEPURATIVE: Purifies the blood

DETERGENT: Cleansing to boils, ulcers, and wounds

DIAPHORETIC: Produces perspiration

DISCUTIENT: Dissolves and removes tumors

DIURETIC: Increases the secretion and flow of urine

EMETIC: Produces vomiting

EMMENAGOGUE: Promotes menstruation

EMOLLIENT: Softening and soothing to inflamed parts

ESCULENT: Eatable as food

EXANTHEMATOUS: Remedy for skin eruptions and diseases

EXPECTORANT: Facilitates expectoration

FEBRIFUGE: Abates and reduces fevers

HEPATIC: Remedy for diseases of the liver

HERPATIG: Remedy for skin eruptions, ringworm, etc.

LAXATIVE: Promotes bowel action

LITHONTRYPTIC: Dissolves calculi in the urinary organs

MATURATING: Ripens or brings boils, tumors, and ulcers to a head

MUCILAGINOUS: Soothing to inflamed parts

NAUSEANT: Produces vomiting

NERVINE: Acts specifically on the nervous system

OPHTHALMICUM: A remedy for disease of the eye

PARTURIENT: Induces and promotes labor at childbirth

PECTORAL: Remedy to relieve chest or lung afflictions

REFRIGERANT: Cooling

RESOLVENT: Dissolves and removes tumors

RUBIFACIENT: Increases circulation, produces red skin

SEDATIVE: Tonic on nerves, also quieting

SIALAGOGUE: Increases the secretion of saliva

STOMACHIC: Strengthens and gives tone to the stomach

STYPTIC: Arrests hemorrhage and bleeding

SUDORIFIC: Produces profuse perspiration

TONIC: Remedy which is invigorating and strengthening

VERMIFUGE: Expels worms

Tonics

A tonic is an agent that is used to give strength to the system. It is always good to take tonic herbs when convalescing from any disease or ailment. The following are all tonic herbs.

White pond lily, boneset, ginger root, capsicum, bitter root, balmony, poplar bark, golden seal, white willow, black horehound, broom, centaury, comfrey, cudweed, ground ivy, elecampane, dandelion, valerian, meadow sweet, mistletoe, mugwort, wood betony, self heal, agrimony, sanicle, skullcap, red raspberry leaves, yarrow, sage, and vervain.

Specific Nerve Tonics: Golden seal is a pure tonic to nervous systems and mucous membranes. It acts as a powerful cleanser to all the mucous membranes in the system.

White willow, Skullcap, Valerian, Mistletoe, Wood Betony, Agrimony and Self Heal are all excellent for nervous tremors.

Tonic for Lungs: One teaspoonful equal parts of the following: comfrey, black horehound, cudweed, ground ivy, elecampane, ginger root, and one-half teaspoon of cayenne is reported to have had soothing effects to the lungs.

Tonics for General Debility and Loss of Appetite: Centaury, dandelion, ground ivy, meadow sweet, mugwort, wood betony, self heal, agrimony, capsicum, balmony, poplar bark, black horehound, broom, sanicle, yarrow, and sage.

Different herbologists recommend varying amounts and recipes to achieve the desired effect of different herbs. Often, one source does not agree with another source on the exact method or amounts to prepare the herbs for human use. Therefore, rather than giving the dosage for each herb, we suggest that you discuss this with the herbologist or chemists from whom you purchase your herbs. Any herbs which are purchased through the mails must state the exact method of preparing it for human use. There are probably thousands of general practitioners across this country who are knowledgeable in the use and preparation of herbs.

Most of the more popular and readily available herbs are sold with directions for their usage right on the label of the box or package. If, however, you are still in doubt as to the exact amounts for your own needs, consult your doctor, *never* try to prescribe for yourself.

Again let us state that *no* herb can be considered a *cure* for any given ailment, by itself. They have, however, been known to have varying degrees of benefit in helping arrest or improve various ailments.

Should you have a particular ailment which you are going to try and treat with herb therapy, you *must* consult your doctor first. Never undertake such a program by yourself. HERBS, IF NOT USED IN THE PROPER MANNER, CAN BE HARMFUL!

In researching the material for this comprehensive chapter on herbs, we found certain books and manuals of great use and would recommend them for the casual or inquisitive reader on the subject of herbs. They are:

Modern Encyclopedia of Herbs, J. M. Kadans, M.D., PhD. Parker Pub.

Eat the Weeds, B. C. Hasris, Barre Publishers

Herbal Manual, H. Ward, L. N. Fowler & Co. Ltd.

The Healing Power of Herbs, Mary Bathel, Wilshire Books

Back to Eden, J. Kloss, Longview Publishing House

Natural & Folk Remedies, C. Wade, Parker Publisher

Ginseng and Other Medicinal Plants, A. R. Harding, A. R. Harding Pub.

Materia Medica and Pharmacology, Culbreth,
Lea & Febiger Pub.

God-Given Herbs for the Healing of Mankind,
W. K. McGrath, McGrath Pub.

The Place of Herbs in Rational Therapy, E.
Robinson, E. Robinson Pub.

Herbs

ABSCESS ROOT: Also known as American Greek
Valerian, False Jacob's Ladder, Sweatroot. Botanical name: *Polemonium retans.* This herb
has a stimulating effect upon glands so as to produce considerable perspiration. It has been recommended for various lung diseases, coughs,
colds and bronchial disturbances.

ACACIA: Also known as Gum Arabic, Egyptian
Thorn, Gum Acacia, Tamarisk Catechu. Botanical names: *Acacia senegal, Acacia arabica,
vera, decurrens.* Habitat: Northern Africa,
Egypt and Middle-east. The gum has a soothing
or softening effect upon the skin or mucous
membrane to which it is applied. It also has an
astringent effect, contracting and hardening
tissues so as to limit secretion of glands. Acacia
is also said to have nutritive qualities, nourishing tissues to which it is applied. Due to its
high tannic acid content, widely known for use
in treatment of burns, acacia may be applied to
burned areas, preventing air from contacting
the burn, and preventing blistering.

ACONITE: Also known as Monkshood, Wolfsbane,

Cuckoo's Cap, Blue Rocket, Friar's Cap, Jacob's Chariot. Botanical name: *Aconitum napellus*. The effect of this herb is that of a sedative or depressant. It has also been used to reduce pain and fever and helps in combating inflammation of the stomach (gastritis), nerve pains of the face (facial neuralgia), inflammation of the mucous membrane (catarrh), ulcerated tonsils, croup and heart spasm.

ACORN: This is the fruit of the Oak tree. Botanical name: *Quercus robur*. The acorn tends to contract and harden tissues and to limit secretion action by the glands. This astringent action has made the mixture applicable for treatment of diarrhea.

ADDER'S TONGUE: Also known as Serpent's Tongue, Dog's Tooth Violet, Yellow Snowdrop, Rattlesnake Violet, Yellow Snakeleaf. Botanical names: *Erythronium americanum* and *Ophioglossum vulgatum*. Habitat: United States. When swallowed, it will cause vomiting and so is an emetic. When placed directly upon tissue, it has a soothing and softening effect and so it is also an emollient. Another reported use for this herb is for the relief of swelling due to accumulation of fluid in various body cavities known as dropsy.

ADRUE: Also known as Guinea Rush. Botanical name: *Cyperus articulatus*. The aroma of this herb tends to reduce the desire for vomiting and is therefore recommended in conditions where it is desired that a person retain the food taken. This herb also acts as a sedative.

AGAR: Also known as Agar-Agar, Japanese Isinglass, Vegetable Gelatin. Botanical names: *Gelidium amansii, Gelidium corneum* of the family Gelidaceae. Habitat: In Japan, Yellow and China Seas, along the eastern coast of Asia, and in the Pacific Ocean. This is an algae which has been used to soothe and relieve inflammation. It has also been used as a mild laxative when mixed in mineral oil.

AGARIC: Also known as White Agaric, Larch, and Purging Agaric. Botanical names: *Polyporus officinalis, Boletus laricis.* This herb will limit secretions of mucous membranes and glands, thus producing an astringent effect. When taken internally, the effect upon the bowels has produced a cleansing result and is therefore also a purgative.

AGRIMONY: Also known as Stickwort, Cocklebur. Botanical name: *Agrimonia eupatoria.* Habitat: Europe. This herb has an astringent effect, as it contracts and hardens tissue. When absorbed into the system, it also strengthens and tones the muscles and is therefore a tonic. This herb also affects the cells of the kidneys, allowing fluids to pass more readily through the kidneys, and is therefore also a diuretic. It can reduce or remove diarrhea. It can also be used to improve the stomach, liver and bowels and assist in the treatment of stones and gravel in the kidneys. It has been used as a gargle for reducing soreness of the mouth and throat.

ALDER, BLACK, AMERICAN: Botanical name: *Prinos verticillatus*. The bark of this tree, when steeped in hot water, produces a solution that has a strong laxative effect.

ALDER, ENGLISH: Botanical name: *Alnus glutinosa*. The leaves are useful when applied to inflamed parts of the body. The bark also produces a mixture which has been used as a tonic and as a gargle for sore throats. It has also been recommended as an astringent, as it tends to contract tissue and reduce secretion of fluids.

ALKANET: Also known as Dyer's Bugloss, Spanish Bugloss, Anchusa, Orchanet. Botanical names: *Alkanna tinctoria, Lithospermum tinctorium, Anchusa tinctoria*. This herb is an emollient. It also has the effect of contracting tissue and causing a cessation of the flow of body liquids. It can be used as an antiseptic for treatment of wounds and when taken internally, it has also destroyed body worms.

ALFALFA: Also known as Buffalo Herb, Sweet Lucerne. Alfalfa is one of the richest land-grown sources of sub-nutritional trace minerals. Most plants are shallow surface feeders. Alfalfa is very high in iron, magnesium, phosphorus, sulphur, sodium, potassium, chlorine and silicon. It is very potent in plant calcium. It is also high in vitamin K, which is so essential to the clotting of blood. It contains eight known enzymes, all of which are necessary to make foods assimilable by the body. It is a good blood builder, good for teeth and bones and inflamed bladder. It helps to produce milk for nursing mothers and aids in the elimination of various drug poisons from the body. In its total effect, it is one of the all-round best herbs in nature.

ALL-HEAL: Also known as Wound-Wort. Botanical name: *Brunella vulgaris*. This European herb has antiseptic qualities and can also help to relieve muscular spasms. It has also been used to assist in starting menstrual flow when irregularities occur.

ALLSPICE: Also known as Pimento, Jamaica Pepper. Botanical name: *Pimenta officinalis*. This herb is an aromatic. It is also a stomachic in that it excites activity in the stomach. It is a carminative in that it tends to remove gases from the upper intestinal tract. Inasmuch as it imparts flavor to almost any food, it is also a condiment. It has been used in cases of diarrhea.

ALOES: Also known as Bombay Aloes; Turkey, Mocha, Zanzibar, Socotrine, Curacao, Bitter, and Cape Aloe. Botanical name: Liliacae family; *Aloe socotrina*. It acts as a cathartic, stomachic, aromatic, emmenagogue, drastic. This is reportedly one of the best herbs to clean out the colon and promote menstruation when suppressed. It helps to clean morbid matter from the stomach, liver, kidneys, spleen and bladder. It has been used for burns, radiation burns, cuts and bruises. It is reportedly very soothing to the stomach and can be used in any case where a laxative is needed.

ALSTONIA BARK: Also known as Fever Bark, Australian Quinine, Australian Febrifuge. Botanical name: *Alstonia constricta*. This can act as an agent and tonic for reducing fever. It has also been effective in some forms of rheumatism.

ALTHEA: Also known as Mallow family, Marshmallow. Botanical name: *Althea officinalis*. This herb acts as demulcent, emollient and pain-soother. It has been used as a douche for irritation of the vagina, bathing inflamed eyes, in making poultices and for irritative diarrhea or dysentery.

AMARANTH: Also known as Red Cockscomb, Love-lies-bleeding. Botanical names: *Amaranthus hypochondriacus, Amaranthus melancholicus*. This herb is an astringent, having the effect of contracting tissue and limiting secretion of glands. It is helpful for excessive bleeding during the menstrual period and is reportedly good for stopping diarrhea as well as bleeding from the bowels. The liquid is also useful as a wash for ulcers and sores and as a gargle for the throat and mouth.

AMMONIACUM: Also known as Persian Gum Ammoniacum. Botanical name: *Dorema ammoniacum*. This is a gum resin that is a natural exudation from the plant and serves as a stimulant, causing removal of secretions of the bronchial passages. It has been used for use in asthmatic conditions involving spasms of the bronchial passages.

ANGELICA, EUROPEAN: Also known as Garden Angelica. Botanical name: *Angelica archangelica*. This herb acts as a stimulant, carminative, emmenagogue, tonic, aromatic, diaphoretic, diuretic, and expectorant. This has been used as a tonic for the stomach, heartburn, gas, colic, colds and fever. This herb has reportedly been found to be valuable in various lung diseases including coughs and shortness of breath. It also has the effect of opening passages in the liver and spleen. Due to this herb's unique ability to clear tiny passages, it has been used to relieve dimness of vision and hearing by placing drops of the fluid into the eyes and ears. It is reported that it heals ulcers and helps restore the normal tissues.

ANGOSTURA: Also known as Cusparia Bark. Botanical names: *Cusparia febrifuga, Galipea officinalis, Bonplandia trifoliata, Galipea cusparia*. This native plant of Venezuela is a tonic and an aromatic. It stimulates functional body activity and has been used for diarrhea, intermittent fevers and for conditions where there has been an accumulation of water in the tissues and cavities.

ANISE: Also known as Anise Seed, Sweet Cumin and Anisum. Botanical name: *Pimpinella anisum Linne*. This acts as a stimulant, aromatic, diaphoretic, relaxant, tonic, carminative and stomachic. This is one of the old herbs, and has many valuable properties. It has helped to prevent fermentation and gas in the stomach and bowels. It is reportedly a good stomach remedy for overcoming nausea and colic.

ARBUTUS, TRAILING: Also known as Gravel Plant, Ground Laurel, Mountain Pink, Winter Pink, Mayflower. Botanical name: *Epigae repens.* This herb is an astringent in that it has the effect of contracting and hardening tissue and checking secretions of mucous membranes. It has reportedly helped persons who have weak bladders or bladders containing so-called gravel or crystalline dust, which are often called bladder stones. It has also been helpful when the urine contains blood or pus.

ARECA NUT: Also known as Betel Nut. Botanical name: *Areca catechu.* This herb contracts and hardens tissue and checks secretions of mucous membranes, and is thus an astringent.

ARENARIA RUBRA: Also known as Sandwort. Botanical names: *Lepigonum rubrum, Tissa rubra, Buda rubra.* This herb acts as a diuretic, stimulating functioning of the bladder. It has been used for inflammation of the bladder, known as cystitis, as well as for bladder stones.

ARNICA: Also known as Leopard's Bane. Botanical name: *Arnica montana.* This herb is used for bruises, strains, sprains, pain, muscular rheumatism, externally in liniments. When taken internally it is reportedly effective as a sedative for the nerves, lessening the irritability of nerves and increasing nerve energy. It has been used for cases of hysteria or high nerve tension. It can reportedly also be used effectively in connection with stimulation of the menstrual function due to obstructions in the flow.

ARROWROOT: Also known as Bermuda Arrowroot. Botanical name: *Maranta arundinacea*. This herb is used as a nutritive drink for infants and convalescents. It also has had a soothing and softening effect upon mucous membranes, in addition to being nutritious.

ASAFETIDA: Also known as Gum Asafetida, Devil's Dung, Food of the Gods. Botanical name: *Umbelliferae, Ferula foetida Regel*. This herb, which is found only in Iran, India and Afghanistan, is a stimulant due to its effect on the brain and nervous system. It is also an expectorant, tonic, laxative, diuretic (urine producing), diaphoretic (produces perspiration), emmenagogue (stimulates menstrual flow), anthelmintic (expels putrified matter from the intestinal tract) and has been reported to have a stimulating effect on the sexual glands. It has been found valuable in cases of excessive air in the stomach of infants, known as colic. It has been helpful to persons who suffer from stomach irritation, hysteria and spasmodic nervous conditions.

ASARABACCA: Also known as Hazelwort, Wild

Nard. Botanical name: *Asarum europaeum*. This herb has been used as an emetic, inducing vomiting, and has also been used as a purgative in cleansing the intestinal tract.

ASH: Also known as Common Ash, Weeping Ash. Botanical name: *Fraxinus excelsior*. This herb has been used as a laxative as well as for general relief from arthritis and rheumatism.

ASPARAGUS: Botanical name: *Asparagus officinalis*. This commonly used plant also contains special healing properties. It has been used as a diuretic for stimulation of action of the kidneys, and as a mild laxative and sedative for the nervous system. It has reportedly been recommended for persons who suffer from enlarged heart and for conditions involving accumulation to an excessive degree of fluids in tissues and in body cavities.

AVENS: Also known as Colewort, Herb Bennet. Botanical names: *Geum urbanum, Radix caryophyllata*. This herb has an astringent effect, in that it checks secretions of the mucous membranes and contracts and hardens tissue. It has been used for its effect in contracting blood vessels so as to stop hemorrhages, thus having a styptic effect. It is also a tonic as it has been reported to have restored power and strength in cases of weakness and debility. It has also been used in cases of diarrhea, as it tends to diminish constant watery discharges from the intestines.

AZADIRACHTA: Also known as Nim, Margosa,

Neem. Botanical name: *Melia azadirachta*. This herb is well known for its use in relieving intestinal worms (anthelmintic) as well as a purgative.

BAEL: Also known as Bel, Indian Bael, Bengal Quince. Botanical name: *Aegle marmelos*. This herb has the effect of contracting tissue and reducing the flow of liquids or fluids from the glands. It is also used in cases of diarrhea and it is reported as non-constipating. It has been recommended for other ailments where there is inflammation of mucous membrane accompanied by ulcers or fever.

BALM OF GILEAD: Botanical name: *Populus balsamifera* or *candicans*. This herb stimulates the ily Labiatae. This herb acts as a diaphoretic, carminative, febrifuge, stimulant and tonic. It has been used in cases of feverish colds, and for relieving headaches. When taken cold, it reportedly relieves fever; when taken hot, it promotes perspiration. It has also been used for painful or suppressed menstruation. It is often used to aid digestion and for relief of nausea and vomiting.

BALM OF GILLEAD: Botanical name: *Populus balsamifera* or *candicans*. This herb stimulates the body organs and also has nutritive value, therefore being both a stimulant and a tonic. It has been used for ailments of the chest, lungs, stomach and kidneys. The ointment has also been found useful for relieving the pains of rheumatism and the gout.

BALMONY: Also known as Bitter Herb, Snake Head, Turtle Bloom. Botanical name: *Chelone glabra*. This herb has many uses. It is a tonic, giving strength to the tissues; it is an anthelmintic, helping to relieve the intestinal tract of morbid matter; it is a detergent, in that it cleanses harmful bacteria from the vital organs; and it is antibilious, being used for disordered conditions of the liver that cause constipation, headache, loss of appetite and vomiting. It also increases the gastric and salivary secretions, and stimulates the appetite. It has been used for sores and eczema.

BAMBOO BRIER: Also known as Wild Sarsaparilla. Botanical name: *Aralia nudicaulis*. This herb is used as an alterative, that is, it alters the processes of nutrition and excretion, restoring the normal functions of the system. It has a tonic effect, increasing the strength and tone of body tissue, and is used in cases of rheumatism and diseases of the skin. It is also used as a blood purifier.

BARBERRY: Also known as Berberis, Oregongrape Root, Trailing Mahonia, Rocky Mountain Grape. Botanical name: *Berberis linne; Berberis vulgaris; Berberis aquifolium*. This herb acts as an astringent, a tonic and stomach aid. It also has alterative qualities, changing nutritive processes to a normal state. It has been used for relief of pain, soreness and burning sensations along the biliary ducts as well as the urinary tracts.

BARLEY: Also known as Pearl Barley, Perlatum. Botanical name: *Hordeum distichon,* of the family Graminaceae. Barley is a nutritive food, containing protein, starch, enzymes and vitamins, and is therefore a valuable food for the sick and convalescent. In addition, this food is soothing to irritated surfaces and can be easily digested. It can also be used for diarrhea or inflammatory conditions of the bowels or other inflammatory conditions of mucous membranes of the body.

BASIL: Also known as Common Basil, Sweet Basil. Botanical name: *Ocium basilicum.* This herb acts as a stimulant, condiment, nervine, aromatic. It is commonly used on areas of the skin that are swollen from insect bites or ivy poison. It also allays excessive vomiting and is effective in aiding digestion.

BAYBERRY: Also known as Bayberry Bush, Myrtle, Tallow Shrub, Vegetable Tallow. Botanical name: *Myrica cerifera.* This herb is used as an astringent, tonic and stimulant. This is one of the most useful herbs. The tea has been used as a gargle for sore throat and to aid in cleansing the throat of all putrid matter. It has restored the mucous secretions to normal activity and cleansed the stomach. It can be used as an emetic after narcotic poisoning of any kind, and it is good to follow with a lobelia emetic. It has been used for all varieties of hemorrhages, whether from the stomach, lungs, uterus, or bowels. It is reportedly ussd to check profuse menstruation and in cases of leucorrhea. It is one of the best herbs for the female organs, also has an excellent effect on the uterus in pregnancy, and makes a good douche.

In case of gangrenous sores, boils, carbuncles, it has been used as a wash and poultice. It also is beneficial to spongy and bleeding gums. Bayberry has been used in treatment of adenoids and catarrh.

BAY LEAVES: Also known as Bay Tree, Indian Bay, Bay Laurel. Botanical name: *Laurus nobilis*. A pleasant tonic, which gives tone and strength to the digestive organs. It expels wind from the stomach and bowels and has been used for cramps.

BEECH: Also known as Beech Tree, Beech Nut Tree. Botanical name: *Fagus ferruginea*. This herb has been used as a tonic, astringent, and antiseptic. It has been known to improve appetite and to aid the softening and healing of wounds and ulcers. Reportedly used in diabetes, internal ulcers, skin diseases, dyspepsia. It is also used for ailments of the liver, kidneys and bladder.

BEARSFOOT, AMERICAN: Also known as Uvedalia, Leaf Cup. Botanical name: *Polymnia uvedalia*. This herb acts to stimulate the glands of the body and produces a laxative effect as well as a pain relieving effect, serving as an anodyne. It has also been reported to have helped cases of liver and spleen congestive conditions. It also aids in digestive conditions known as dyspepsia, especially hepatic dyspepsia, resulting from liver disease.

BELLADONNA: Also known as Deadly Nightshade, Dwale, Black Cherry Root. Botanical name: *Atropa belladonna*. This herb serves as a diuretic, increasing the secretion of urine. It also serves as an anodyne relieving pain, and relaxes overcontracted smooth muscle and is therefore a sedative. It depresses sensory nerve endings. Its action also makes it effective in the condition involving loss of semen involuntarily, known as spermatorrhea. Despite its sedative action, it helps stimulate the circulation.

BENNE: Also known as Sesam, Gingelly, Sesame. Botanical name: *Sesamum indicum*. The leaves and seeds of this herb are used as a demulcent and as a laxative. This herb, in its tea form, has been used in various ophthalmic complaints, such as inflammation or soreness.

BENZOIN: Botanical name: *Styrax benzoin, Styrax benzoin dryander, Styrax tonkinensis*. Also called Benjamin tree, benzoin laurel, gum Benjamin, gum benzoin, palembang benzoin, siam benzoin, sumatra benzoin. A dry powder is prepared from the sap of this herb, and a tincture made with alcohol. An expectorant, it is useful in treating coughs and bronchitis and often used in cough medicines. Used externally it helps relieve wounds and sores. It also acts as an antiseptic and a stimulant.

BERBERIS: Botanical name: *Berberis vulgaris.* Also Barberry. The Egyptians used this bitter tonic for treating fevers, and the American Indians ate the berries in a jelly or jam and as a tonic for liver ailments. During the 19th century it was used in New England as a medicine for consumptives. Its action is similar to that of Golden Seal and it is used in the same way.

BETHROOT: Botanical name: *Trillium pendulum* and *trillium erectum.* Also Birth-root, Dough Root, Ground Lily, Indian Shamrock, Jew's Harp, Lamb's Quarters, Milk Ipecac, Three-Leaved Nightshade, Trillium, Wakerobin. Besides acting as a tonic and alterative, this herb helps as a pectoral in treatment of bronchial troubles, coughs, lung hemorrhages and pulmonary consumption. It reportedly is used to stem excessive menstruation and as a douche for leucorrhea and other vaginal problems. In an enema, bethroot soothes rectal irritations; the herb is also used for diarrhea and dysentery.

BILBERRIES: Botanical name: *Vaccinum myrtillus.* Also Huckleberries, Whortleberries, Hurtle berries. This herb has been valuable during typhoid epidemics both as a preventative and as a treatment. A tea from the dried berries relieves dropsy and kidney or bladder stones, and has been used for diarrhea and bowel derangements. It also may serve as an enema, a diuretic, a gargle for sore throats and as an astringent for wounds. The ripe fruit reportedly relieves fever and quenches thirst, and the leaves yield a substance known as Myrtillin, which helps reduce blood sugar as does insulin.

BIRCH: Botanical name: *Betula alba*. Also known as White Birch. A bitter, this herb increases the tone of the gastro-intestinal mucous membrane and produces an oil (from the bark), Oleum Rusci, which is used in the relief of gonorrhea and skin diseases such as eczema.

BIRTHWORT: *Aristolochia longa*. Besides its aromatic properties, birthworth has been successful in relieving the symptoms of gout and rheumatism because it is a stimulant for both circulation and glandular functions.

BISTORT: Botanical name: *Polygonum bistorta*. Also called Adderwort, Dragonwort, Easter Giant, Patience Dock, Red Legs, Snake Weed, Sweet Dock. This herb acts as a powerful astringent and had been used in cases of cholera, diarrhea, dysentery and leucorrhea and as a wash for sores on the mouth or gums, as well as external open or running sores (i.e. smallpox, measles, pimples, insect stings, snake bites). Powdered, it is a styptic and will stop bleeding when applied to a wound. It reportedly decreases or regulates menstrual flow when used in a douche. It is also a diuretic and alterative.

BITTERROOT: *Apocynum* and *rosaemifolium*. Also

called Catchfly, Dogsbane, Flytrap, Honey Bloom, Milk Ipecac, Milkweed, Wandering Milkweed, Western Wallflower. The root of this plant seems to have an excellent effect on the liver, kidneys and bowels and can aid in digestion and help to expel worms. It has also been used in treating diabetes and diseases of the joints and mucous membranes such as rheumatism and neuralgia. It has been known to rid the system of impurities (i.e. gallstones) and to remedy fevers of various kinds.

BITTERSWEET: *Solanum dulcamara.* Common names are Fever Twig, Felenwort, Garden Nightshade, Nightshade, Nightshade Vine, Scarlet Berry, Staff Vine, Violet Bloom, Wolf Grape. A soothing anodyne when used externally, this is also an hepatic used as a salve or ointment either by itself (in leprosy), with yellowdock (for skin diseases and sores), or with camomile (for bruises, sprains and corns). It will also purify the blood, make the kidneys and other glandular organs active and increase menstrual flow. Thus it is a deobstruent and aperient or laxative as well. It is also used as a resolvent.

BITTERSWEET, AMERICAN: *Celastrus scandens.* Also False Bittersweet, Waxwort. This alterative acts, also, as a diuretic, thereby aiding in normal functioning of the liver. It has been found helpful in treating leucorrhea and in bringing about delayed menstruation. Perspiration may be induced by drinking the tea.

BLACKBERRY: *Rubus villosus,* of the Rose family, Rosaceae. Also known as Bramble, Rubus, Dewberry, Gout Berry, Cloud Berry, Rudi Fructus. Having both an astringent and a tonic effect, this plant has been highly esteemed in relieving diarrhea. An invigorating tonic and gargle.

BLACK COHOSH: *Cimicifuga racemosa.* Also called Black Snake Root, Bugbane, Bugwort, Rattleroot, Rattlesnake's Root, Rattleweed, Rich Weed, Squaw Root. This herb acts as a nervine and antispasmodic. As such is used in cases of hysteria, St. Vitus's Dance (chorea), epilepsy, and convulsions. It has been known to be an effective pain reliever in childbirth. It has been used for dropsy, rheumatism, meningitis, asthma (it is an astringent and expectorant), delirium tremens and snake and insect bites. As a syrup it quiets coughs and soothes liver and kidney troubles. It is also an emmenagogue, alterative and diaphoretic.

BLACK CURRANT: *Ribes nigrum.* Besides the nutritive value of the fruit, this plant's leaves are a diuretic and have been used as a tonic and for hoarseness, cleansing wounds and ulcers, and to reduce fever. The juice is an antiseptic and blood purifier, thereby of value in anemia, malnutrition and general debility.

BLACK HAW: *Viburnum rufidulum rafinesque.* Also American Sloe, Stagbush, and *Viburnum Prunifolium.* Reportedly the principal use of this herb is during pregnancy for nervous disorders, pain relief, and to prevent miscarriages. It is also used as a uterine astringent to draw together the soft tissue and prevent painful menstruation. It has also been used to check uterine bleeding.

BLACK WILLOW BARK: *Salix nigra, Salix discolor.* Commonly called Calkins Willow, Marsh, Pussy Willow. This astringent and antiseptic has been used as a douche to relieve inflamed and ulcerated surfaces of mucous membrane of the vagina and for relief of ovarian pain. It is a treatment for nocturnal involuntary emissions and a depressant for the sexual glands where irritation of the sexual organs results from genito-urinary problems. In powdered form the bark has been known to relieve inactive ulcers or gangrene. The herb is also effective for rheumatism and inflammation of the joints, muscles and nerves.

BLOODROOT: *Sanguinaria canadensis.* Also Indiana Plant, Pauson, Red Paint Root, Red Root, Red Puccoon. In small doses bloodroot stimulates the heart and digestive organs; a large dose acts as a sedative. It is effective in speeding the process of healing of piles and nasal tumors (and American Thomasonians use it to treat adenoids) , sores and diseases of the skin; and as a relief for chest diseases such as coughs, colds, bronchitis, pneumonia.

BLUE COHOSH: *Caulophyllum thalictroides.* Also Blue Berry, Blue or Yellow Ginseng, Papoose

Root, Squaw Root. A most valuable herb to women, it is used in chronic uterine problems, leucorrhea, vaginitis and cramps. American Indians use it to facilitate childbirth and induce labor. As an emmenagogue it is also used to regulate menstruation. It has been used for dropsy, colic, hysteria, heart palpitations and high blood pressure and diabetes. It has been reported to soothe hiccoughs and other spasms such as epilepsy and whooping cough. It contains the minerals potassium, magnesium, calcium, iron, silicon and phosphorus which help to alkalinize the blood and urine.

BLUE FLAG: *Iris versicolor.* Also Flag Iris, Flag Lily, Fleur-de-lis, Flower-de-luce, Iris, Liver Lily, Poison Flag, Snake Lily, Water Flag, Water Lily. This herb was used before the discovery of penicillin in curing syphilis. For liver troubles, it increases the flow of urine (diuretic action), thereby eliminating poisons from the blood and relieving indigestion and its accompanying dizziness and headaches. It is also a laxative and vermifuge. The powdered herb will induce sneezing to clear nasal passages or, if applied to a wound, will speed healing. It is also a remedy for insect bites and stings. The juice reportedly relieves hemorrhoids and is relaxing and stimulating.

BLUE MALLOW: *Malva sylvestris.* Also called Cheese Flower, Common mallow, Mauls. A drink prepared by pouring boiling water over the herb has been found to be popular for coughs, colds and similar ailments. It will also soothe and soften the skin when it is applied directly to the body part in powder form.

BLUE VIOLET: *Viola cuculata.* Also Common Blue Violet and Violet. Among those ailments said to have been remedied by the leaves of this plant are tumors, gout, coughs, colds, sore throat, sores, ulcers, cancer scrofula, syphilis, bronchitis, and difficult breathing due to gases and morbid matter in the stomach and bowels. It also relieves internal ulcers and as a mucilaginous herb soothes headache and head congestion and whooping cough. Combined with nerveroot, skullcap, or black cohosh it serves as a soothing nervine. It is also a laxative, and emetic and an alterative.

BOLDO: *Peumus boldus.* Sometimes called Boldea, Boldu, or Fragrans. This herb is a native of Chile and its leaves are imported for use in the treatment of various disturbances. It stimulates the secretion and excretion of urine, serving as a diuretic, and is therefore used in chronic hepatic torpor. An antiseptic as well, it prevents the growth of microorganisms and has been reported to be effective in cases of inflammation of the bladder and ridding the urinary tract of gonorrhea germs.

BONESET: *Eupatorium perfoliatum.* Common names are Indian Sage, Thoroughwort. It is both a febrifuge and an expectorant and provides relief for coughing spells and catarrh. It may also be used as an ointment for some skin diseases.

BORAGE: *Borago officinalis.* Burrage or Common Bugloss. The tea is used to bathe sore, inflamed eyes. Taken internally, the tea cleanses the blood by diuretic action and is effective for fevers, yellow jaundice, to expel poisons of all kinds due to snake bites, insect bites. It has been known to strengthen the heart and is used for coughs; it soothes itch, ringworms, tetters, scabs, sores, ulcers and, as a gargle, ulcers in the mouth and throat.

BOX LEAVES: *Buxus sempervirens.* This herb, acting as a depurative, is helpful in curing yellow jaundice. It may be made into a tea or swallowed directly, and is used as a tonic for general weakness or debility.

BROOM: *Cytisus scoparius.* Also Irish Broom. The leaves and stem are used with uva ursi, cleavers and dandelion as a diuretic to cleanse the kidneys and bladder. It may also be used internally to relieve toothache, dropsy, ague and gout. Externally it may be made into an ointment for lice or vermin. It contains potash.

BRYONY: *Tamus communis, Linn.* Sometimes Black Bryony, Blackeye Root, Bryonia, English Mandrake, Mandragora. A pulp made from the root of this plant is rubbed into areas of the body affected by rheumatism, gout or paralysis. Bruises and discolorations as well as freckles also seem to be removed by this procedure (thus the name "blackeye" root). A tincture prepared from the herb will act as a diuretic; it has also been used for accumulation of fluid in body cavities or tissues and for coughs, influenza, bronchitis. It is also reported to heal sunburn and effectively cleanse ulcers on the skin and is used in malarial and zymotic diseases.

BUCHU: *Barosma betulina.* Common names are Bookoo, Bucku, Buku, Thumb, Diosma. Used as a tincture or as a tea, buchu is reported to be one of the best aids for urinary problems. Taken warm it produces perspiration and soothes leucorrhea and enlargement of the prostate gland and irritation of the urethra. It has also been used successfully for rheumatism and dropsy and in the early stages of diabetes.

BUCKBEAN: *Menyanthes trifoliata.* Also Bitter Trefoil, Bitterworm, Bog Bean, Bog Myrtle, Brook Bean, Marsh Clover, Marsh Trefoil, Water Shamrock. Buckbean seems to be especially effective in cases of stomach complaints. It is used to treat dyspepsia and stomach catarrh, and to promote digestion. Taken in large doses it is emetic and anthelmintic. A tonic and bitter, it is also used to relieve rheumatism, scrofula, scurvy, jaundice and other liver troubles, and intermittent fevers.

BUCKTHORN BARK: *Rhamnus frangula.* Sometimes called Alder Buckthorn, Black Alder Dogwood, Black Alder Tree, Black Dogwood, European Black Alder, European Buckthorn, Persian Berries. Taken internally, the bark of the buck-thorn seems to relieve constipation and keep the bowels regular. (The fruit is a purgative.) It has been used for gout, dropsy and skin diseases and, taken hot, produces profuse perspiration. An ointment of the herb provides relief from itching and has been reported to be helpful in the removal of warts.

BUGLE: *Ajuga reptans.* Sometimes known as bu-gula. This aromatic herb is a tonic which tones the gastrointestinal mucous membrane. It is also an astringent and widely used to stop hemor-rhaging and for bile disorders.

BUGLEWEED: *Lycopus virginicus.* Also Sweet Bu-gle, or Water Bugle. This mild narcotic has been used for coughs and to relieve pulmonary bleeding. It has a sedative as well as an astrin-gent effect, tending to contract tissues of the mucous membrane and reduce fluid discharges.

BUGLOSS: *Echium vulgare.* Sometimes called Blue-weed, Viper's Bugloss. The action of this herb is expectorant, diaphoretic, and demulcent, used to reduce fever due to colds and inflamma-tion of the respiratory tract.

BURDOCK: *Arctium lappa.* Bardana, Beggar's But-tons, Burrs, Burr Seed, Clot-bur, Grass Bur-dock, Hardock, Harebur, Hurrburr, Lappa, Turkey Burr Seed. It is the seed of this plant which has medicinal properties. The dried, first-year root is also used. A seed tincture has been found to be a stomachic tonic and has aided in the relief of the chronic skin condition known as psoriasis inveteratar, as well as boils and carbuncles. Applied externally a decoction made from the root is used for gout, rheumatism, scrofula, canker sores, syphilis, sciatica, and gonorrhea. It seems to be one of the best blood purifiers. In the form of a salve or tea it helps relieve swellings, burns and hemorrhoids. The plant produces *inulin* which is used in the production of fructose which has been used in the diet of diabetics.

BURNET: *Pimpinella saxifraga.* Also Burnet Saxifrage, European Burnet, Pimpernel. A stomachic used to cleanse the lungs and stomach. It helps heal cuts, wounds, sores, piles, and relieve tooth and earache. It also has a pleasant odor.

BURR MARIGOLD: *Bidens tripartita.* Also Water Agrimony. This garden or wild plant is astringent, diuretic and diaphoretic and has been recommended for dropsy, gout and hemorrhages of urinary and respiratory organs.

BUTTER-BUR: *Petasites vulgaris, Tussilago, Petasites.* Also Common Butterbur. This valuable herb is a stimulant and diuretic and has been effective in strengthening the cardiac muscles.

BUTTERNUT BARK: *Juglans cinerea.* Also Kisky Thomas Nut, Lemon Walnut, Oilnut, Oilnut Bark, White Walnut. This plant has several medicinal qualities: it is an alterative, anthelmintic, astringent, cathartic and cholagogue. It will also expel intestinal worms and relieve fevers and colds.

CALAMUS: *Acorus calamus.* Also Grass Myrtle, Myrtle Flag, Sea Sedge, Sweet Cane, Sweet Flag, Sweet Grass, Sweet Myrtle, Sweet Root, Sweet Rush, Sweet Sedge. The root of this plant is especially effective for stomach complaints: it improves gastric juices and keeps the stomach sweet while preventing acids, gases and fermentation in the stomach. It is also good for dyspepsia and increases appetite. It is claimed to destroy the desire for tobacco. A tea of the herb may be applied to burns, sores and ulcers and is valuable in treating scrofula.

CALUMBA: *Jateorhiza calumba.* This root is used for stomach troubles and indigestion in general. It acts as a febrifuge and is a bitter tonic.

CALOTROPIS: *Calotropis procera, asclepias procera.* Sometimes called Mudar Bark. It is reported that the powdered bark mixed with water, olive oil or antiseptic vaseline may be applied directly to the skin for relief of eczema. Taken internally, it has been found beneficial for diarrhea and dysentery.

CAMOMILE: *Anthemis nobilis.* Common names are Chamomile, Ground Apple, Whig Plant. A well-known home remedy, a tea made from the blossoms is an excellent tonic and beneficial in the treatment of many ailments, among them dyspepsia, colds, bronchitis, bladder troubles, ague,

dropsy and jaundice. The tea is a soothing wash
for sore eyes, as well as other sores and wounds.
As a poultice it is used on swellings and pains.
It promotes menstrual flow, softens skin, is effective for colic in infants, intermittent fever,
and the early stages of typhoid. It is good in
hysteria and nervous diseases. It is also a popular table tea. In pulverized form the flower-
heads may be made with soapwort into a shampoo, especially for fair hair.

CAMPHOR: *Cinnamomum camphora, Laurus
camphora, Camphora officinarum.* Sometimes
referred to as Gum Camphor or Laurel Camphor. As an anodyne, it is especially beneficial
in cases of gout, rheumatism and neuralgia, and
is used to relieve irritation of the sexual organs.
Externally it may be applied to inflamed or
bruised areas. Taken internally it is a sedative
and is valuable for colds and their accompanying symptoms. Perspiration may be induced by
ingestion of the herb and fever reduced. Physicians will sometimes use oil of camphor as a
heart stimulant.

CARAWAY: *Carum carui.* Sometimes called Kum-
mel or Caraway Seed. The seeds may be taken
in hot water or milk for colic and colds. It is a
digestive aid, strengthening and toning the
stomach and preventing catarrh on the alimentary tract. The powdered seeds may be made
into a poultice to remove bruises. It is also used

to flavor other herbs and prevent griping, as well as in baking. The root may be eaten as turnips are.

CARDAMOMS: *Elettaria cardamomum*. The seeds of this fruit, taken warm, are an aromatic helpful in flatulence. It is a carminative and a stomachic.

CARROT: *Daucus carota*. Bee's Nest Plant, Bird's Nest Root, arden Carrot, Queen Anne's Lace, Wild Carrot. Both the root and seeds are used. Grated, they make an effective poultice for ulcers, abscesses, carbuncles, scrofulas, cankerous sores and severe wounds. A carrot diet has sometimes relieved bladder, liver and kidney problems. They are used for dropsy, gravel, painful urination, to increase menstrual flow, and expel worms from the bowels. The powdered seeds make a tea which is reported to relieve colic and increase the flow of urine.

CASCARA SAGRADA: *Rhamnus purschiana*. Bear Wood, Bearberry, Bitter Bark, California Buckthorn, Chittam Bark, Coffee Berry Bark, Dogwood Bark, Persian Bark, Purschiana Bark, Sacred Bark. The fresh bark is a powerful gastro-intestinal irritant and emetic sometimes recommended as an intestinal tonic and as for relief of gallstones. It has been used for chronic constipation and digestive disorders, and is not habit forming. It increases the secretion of bile and has been used for liver complaints, especially enlarged liver. Other uses are in gout, dyspepsia, piles and to regulate the bowels.

CASTOR OIL PLANT: *Ricinus communis.* Also Palma Christi. This is a well-known purgative and cathartic which is gentle enough for use by children and pregnant women. Besides being a treatment for constipation, it is effective in colic in infants and in cases of diarrhea resulting from slow digestion. Applied externally the oil tends to soothe itch, ringworm, and cuts on the skin.

CAYENNE: *Capiscum annuum.* Also called Cayenne Pepper, Chili Pepper, African Red Pepper, Spanish Pepper, Bird Pepper, Pod Pepper, Cockspur Pepper, Red Pepper. Red pepper is reportedly one of the best and quickest stimulants among the herbal medicines and also has the advantage of causing no negative side effects: it stimulates the heart but does not increase the blood pressure. It is used as a tonic. It has been used as a healing application for bruises, sprains, wounds, burn and sunburns, and pyorrhea. A plaster of cayenne has been used to relieve internal inflammation most efficaciously and therefore has been used in connection with pleurisy and rheumatism. One author reports that, with an emetic, an enema, sudorifics, and cayenne he has cured cases of rheumatism overnight. The effect of this herb is to equalize circulation, as well as to stimulate the glands, and has been used for ague, spring fever, and in cases of excess mucus in the respiratory passages, as it facilitates expectoration. For its astringent quality, it has been administered for sore throat and diphtheria as a gargle. With bayberry it helps to stop uterine hemorrhages. It has reportedly been used as a remedy for hangover, and for cold feet a small amount may be sprinkled in the socks. To relieve toothache, cotton wool saturated with oil of capiscum has been packed into the tooth, where it acts as a stimulant and an antiseptic. It has none of the irritating effects of black pepper or mustard.

CATNIP: *Nepeta cataria.* Commonly called Cat Mint, Catrup, Cat's Wort, Field Balm. One of the oldest household remedies, it is an antispasmodic and anodyne helpful in convulsions. Further, it reportedly restores menstruation and allays gas or acids in the stomach and bowels. It also prevents griping. Reportedly, an enema is soothing and relaxing and will induce urination when it has stopped. For the treatment of colds, it has reduced fever and produced perspiration. It is also a tonic.

CEDRON: *Simaba cedron.* Sometimes called Rattlesnake's Bones. The tea of this plant has been recommended as a generally invigorating and strengthening drink. It reportedly prevents gas in the stomach and is effective for intermittent fevers. As an antispasmodic it has been used for fits and nervous disorders and any kind of spasm. Externally, a strong tea may be used for snake or insect bites.

CELANDINE: *Chelidonum majus.* Not to be mistaken for Small or Lesser Celandine (Pilewort), this herb has been found helpful for jaundice, eczema and other skin diseases. It may be applied directly to abrasions and bruises and the fresh juice to corns and warts. It is claimed that a decoction of the herb or roots boiled in white wine serves as a deobstruent for liver and bladder.

CELERY: *Apium graveolens.* Also called Smallage. The seeds and the ripe fruit (dried) of this plant have reportedly had an excellent tonic and stimulant effect. They affect the kidneys, producing an increased flow of urine. It has been used in cases of nervousness, neuralgia, and rheumatism. It is also a diaphoretic. The stalks are a popular food and the seeds are a delicious flavoring.

CHICKWEED: *Stelleria media.* Commonly known as Adder's Mouth, Satin Flower, Starwort, Starweed, Stitchwort. This garden pest has multiple healing properties and may be used as a food (prepared like spinach) as well. Reportedly, any form of internal inflammation is soothed and healed by its application: colds and coughs, hoarseness, bronchitis, pleurisy, inflamed bowels. It has been used as a soothing poultice for boils, burns, skin diseases, sore eyes, and wounds. It is said to be one of the best remedies for tumors, piles, swollen testes, ulcerated throat and mouth, and deafness. It may be taken internally for blood poisoning and as a poultice applied externally. A salve of the powder may also be applied, in addition to bathing with the tea. A bath in the tea has been used for sores and skin problems. It is also given to pigs for a disease known as white scour.

CHAULMOOGRA: *Taraktogenos Kurzii.* The powdered seed may be taken or an oil made from the seed may be administered as an ointment or taken internally. A laxative and febrifuge when taken internally, it helps relieve skin eruptions and stiffness of the joints.

CHICORY: *Cichorium endiva.* Blue Sailors, Garden Endive, or Garden Chicory, Endive, Succory. The root of this plant is best known for its use with coffee, but is also effective as a hepatic and for disorders of the urinary canal, stomach and spleen. It has been used to settle an upset stomach by expelling morbid matter, while also toning up the system.

CHERRYLAUREL: *Prunus laurocerasus.* When taken internally, its powdered leaves have been used as a sedative and have often been used to relax the muscles involved in coughing. It has been used for asthma and whooping cough and other diseases involving severe coughing.

CHIRETTA: *Swertia chirata.* Sometimes called Chirayta, Griseb. A bitter tonic. With suitable hepatics and laxatives, it sometimes forms part of a soothing tonic for liver complaints, dyspepsia and constipation.

CINQUEFOIL: *Potentilla reptans.* Also Fivefinger, Five Leaf Grass. When an astringent skin lotion is called for this herb has been applied. It has also been taken as a gargle and internally for diarrhea.

CLEAVERS: *Galium aparine.* Also Bedstraw, Burweed, Catchweed, Cheese Rent Herb, Clabbergrass, Cleaverwort, Clivers, Erriffe, Goose's Hair, Goose Grass, Goose-share, Goosebill, Gravel Grass, Grip Grass, Hayriffe, Milk Sweet, Poor Robin, Savoyan, Scratch Weed. Reportedly, an infusion of this herb is very effective for kidney and bladder problems and may be combined with broom, buchu, gravelroot, marsh mallow, and uvu ursi to act as a diuretic. It seems to dissolve bladder stones. For fever, scarlet fever, and measles its refrigerant and diaphoretic properties are said to be excellent, and it has been used both as a skin cleanser and for skin diseases. As a blood purifier it has been used in connection with gonorrhea and jaundice. Applied to a bleeding wound it reportedly causes clotting and stops bleeding, as well as hastening healing. The oil of the herb may be applied for earache.

CLOVER, RED: *Trifolium pratense.* Also Cleaver Grass, Cow Grass, Marl Grass. This attractive and common flower may be made into a tea for both internal and external use. It may also be combined with blue violet, burdock, yellow dock, dandelion root, rock rose and golden seal to make a concoction for remedy of growths and leprosy. The warm tea has been said to be very soothing to the nerves and therefore has been helpful for spasms and severe coughing. It has been used as a mild stimulant. As a salve it may be applied to wounds.

Gather the blossoms when in full bloom. Dry in the shade and hang in paper bags in a dry place. A tea can then be made from them.

CLOVER, WHITE: *Trifolium repens.* Common names are Melilot, Shamrock, Sweet Lucerne. A salve may be made of the clover blossoms and yellowdock in equal parts. A strong tea applied to external sores helps speed healing, and, taken internally, serves as a cleanser and blood purifier.

CLOVES: *Eugenia aromatica.* Sometimes called Clavos. A powerful carminative, this reportedly relieves gas pain in the stomach and bowel. Because of its stimulant effect, it has improved digestion as well as promoted the flow of saliva and gastric juices. It is an excellent carminative to reduce griping of other herbs. Cloves have been used to relieve pain of toothache, lumbago, rheumatism, muscle cramps and neuralgia.

COFFEE: *Coffea arabica.* In the popular drink, the ground coffee seeds are a diuretic, causing an increase in the activity of the kidneys. It is often used to aid in expelling the effects of alcohol and prevents vomiting by acting as an anti-emetic. The caffeine in coffee is a stimulant and increases the heartbeat. It has also been used to dispel stupor and drowsiness when they are caused by excessive use of narcotics, thus acting as an anti-narcotic. There are also claims that it is helpful for bladder stones, rheumatism and gout.

COLOMBO: *Cocculus palmatus.* A very fine but bitter tonic, this reportedly will strengthen and tone the entire system. It is an antiemetic that can be used in pregnancy and for chronic colon trouble, diarrhea and cholera. It has also been used to improve the appetite.

COLTSFOOT: *Tussilago farfara.* Sometimes called Coughwort, Horsefoot, British Tobacco, Flower Velure, Ginger Root. The leaves of this plant often constitute one ingredient in cough medicines for asthma and whooping cough as they are both pectoral and emollient. It has also been found in medicines for lung ailments such as tuberculosis and catarrh. It has been used in cases of sinusitis, ague, piles, fever and swellings and has been applied externally to scrofulous tumors (or taken internally) or to the lungs and throat. The leaves have also been smoked to soothe the mucous membranes of throat and lungs and relieve congestion of asthma or bronchitis.

COMFREY: *Symphytum officinale.* Also Blackwort, Consolidae, Gum Plant, Healing Herb, Knitback, Knitbone, Nipbone, Slippery Root. This reportedly popular cough remedy has also been taken for arthritis, coughs, catarrh, consumption, excessive expectoration in asthma, sinusitis, and ulceration of the stomach, kidney or bowels. It has been used in cases of bloody urine. To relieve swellings, bruises, sprains and fractures a compress of the hot tea has been applied. It has also helped to relieve the pain. This same treatment reportedly also works on breasts sore from excess milk, headaches, eye injuries, tonsilitis, anal or rectal itching, arthritis or gout, gangrene and burns. As an infusion comfrey has been used to treat female debility, anemia, leucorrhea and gall and liver conditions, diarrhea and pulmonary diseases such as pneumonia. It has been said to be a good general cleanser when taken internally and is reportedly rich in calcium and protein and may be applied to fruit juice for nutritious drink.

CORAL: *Corallorhiza odontorhiza.* Sometimes called Crawley, Chicken's Toes, Dragon's Claw, Fever Root, Turkey Claw. This root has been used for skin diseases, boils, tumors, scrofula, scurvy, menstrual cramps, pleurisy, and is said to be effective for enlarged veins. It acts as a diaphoretic and febrifuge without exciting the system. It is sometimes combined with blue cohosh to produce an emmenagogue.

CORIANDER: *Coriandrum satium.* This pleasant

flavoring strengthens and tones the stomach and acts as a carminative as well. It has also been used to alleviate pain in the bowels caused by laxatives.

CORNSILK: *Zea mays, Stigmata maidis.* Also known as Corn, Maize Jagnog. This is the yellow silk of sweet corn; reportedly used for irritation of the urinary organs and for painful urination caused by stones in the bladder or trouble with the prostate gland. It seems to be an excellent remedy for kidney and bladder troubles, such as enuresis.

COTTON ROOT: *Gossypium herbaceum.* The powdered bark of the root of this herb has been used to bring on retarded menstruation.

COUCHGRASS: *Agropyrum repens.* Sometimes called Twitchgrass or Quick grass. The powdered root of this herb has been used to stimulate activity of the kidneys and bladder and increase the flow of urine. It could therefore be helpful for bladder and urinary problems and a mild purgative. It may be taken for gout and rheumatism and to soothe the mucous membranes.

COWSLIP: *Primula veris.* Also Herb Peter, Paigles, Palsywort. This antispasmodic seems also to be effective in soothing restlessness and insomnia. Cowslip has been used at times for rheumatism, gout and paralysis but its value for these diseases has been disapproved.

CRAMP BARK: *Viburnum opulus.* Guelder rose, High Cranberry, Snowball Tree. In a decoction, this has been used as a nervine and antispasmodic, soothing cramps and other muscular spasms.

CRANESBILL: *Geranium pratense.* As a douche with bistort this has been used for leucorrhea. It reportedly will also stop bleeding, both internal and external, and has been used as an astringent and tonic for the kidneys.

CREEPING JENNY: European Bindweed. The roots of this plant have been said to act very rapidly as a styptic for wounds.

CUBEB BERRIES: *Piper cubeba.* Also Java Pepper, Tailed Cubebs and Tailed Pepper. It has been said that this tasty seasoning can also serve as a tonic for the stomach and bowels, as an aid in bronchial troubles and for chronic bladder troubles. As an aromatic it has been used in gonorrhea and leucorrhea. It is also carminative, a purgative, and a diuretic.

CUDWEED: *Gnaphalium uliginosum.* Also Cotton Weed, or Marsh Cudweed. This herb is an astringent and has been used as a gargle for inflammation of the salivary glands.

CULVER'S ROOT: *Veronicastrum virginicum, Leptandra virginicum.* Also Black Root, Bowman's Root, Culver's Physic, Tall Speedwell, Tall Veronica. The root and rhizome of this plant have been used to treat indigestion resulting from insufficient flow of bile from the liver. When fresh, the root is a strong and rather violent cathartic, and in mild doses it is a tonic.

DAMIANA: *Turnera diffusa*. Sometimes called Turnera. It will reportedly increase the flow of urine, has a mild laxative effect, and has been used as a nerve tonic in cases of physical or mental exhaustion.

DANDELION: *Taraxacum officinale*. Also Blow Ball, Cankerwort, Lion's Tooth, Priest's Crown, Puff Ball, Swine Snout, White Endive. Dandelion greens are used in salads and as a nutritious vegetable. The root may be ground, roasted and prepared as coffee, and it has none of the bad effects of that drink. Prepared this way and drunk regularly it reportedly acts as a mild laxative and diuretic. The sodium salts in the plant should act as blood purifiers. The herb is reportedly useful for dropsy, eczema, scurvy, scrofula, diabetes, inflammation of the bowels, and fevers.

DIGITALIS: *Digitalis pulverata* and *Digitalis purpurea*. Also Cottagers, Dead Men's Bells, Fairy Bells, Fairy Cap, Fairy Fingers, Fairy's Glove, Fairy Thimbles, Flopdock, Foxglove, Folk's Glove, Figwort, Ladies' Glove, Throatwort. A heart toner and stimulant, this herb must be used with the greatest care as it can also cause overstimulation and paralysis. A doctor's direction is strongly recommended. For burns or scalds an ointment made by beating the blossoms into lard is reportedly soothing. The berries contain large amounts of vitamin C.

DEVIL'S BIT: *Scabiosa succisa,* or Ofbit. An infusion of this herb has helped to relieve coughs and fevers.

DILL: *Anethum graveolens.* Sometimes called Eneldo. This popular food seasoning is also used in digestive disorders. It reportedly expels wind from the stomach and bowels and prevents gas and fermentation. It has been used for colic in children. It has been used to soothe pains and swellings, quiet the nerves, and to stop hiccoughs.

ECHINACEA: *Brauneria angustifolia.* Common names are Black Sampson, Cornflower, Kansas Niggerhead, Purple Cove Flower, Red Sunflower, Sampson Root. This reportedly excellent blood purifier has been used in any disease resulting from impurities in the blood, including blood poisoning. It is also said to relieve dyspepsia and gastrointestinal pain, and to be an analgesic. It has also been used as a gargle.

ELDER: *Sambucus nigra.* Elderberry. The flowers of this familiar tree have often been used, with peppermint and yarrow, to reduce fever in colds and as a bath to relieve inflamed eyes. Elderberry wine has been taken for colds and influenza.

ELECAMPANE: *Inula helenium.* Also Aunée or Scabwort. Though a very popular medicine in the seventeenth century, the claims for elecampane have been greatly revised. In combination with other herbs it has been used in cough medicines and for asthma and bronchitis. It is an expectorant and a tonic for the lungs and mucous membranes. It is also an emmenagogue used to bring on menstruation, and reportedly acts to expel kidney and bladder stones and to relieve retention of urine.

ERGOT: *Claviceps purpurea, Secale cornulum.* Also known as Spurred Rye or Smut of Rye. This is the fungus obtained from rye grains. It has been used for dysmenorrhea (painful menstruation) and amenorrhea (abnormal stoppage of menstruation) and leucorrhea (a whitish vaginal discharge). It is also said to be helpful in male disorders such as enlarged prostate and involuntary discharge of semen and in gonorrhea. Another use has been as a styptic for internal bleeding.

ERYNGO: *Eryngium maritimum.* Also Sea Eryngo or Sea Holly. Eryngo root has been used in bladder disorders. It is usually used in combination with other herbs, such as barberry bark or wild carrot.

EUCALYPTUS: *Eucalyptus globulus.* Also Blue Gum Tree. The leaves and oil from this tree are an extremely potent but safe antiseptic. It is also inhaled for sore throat or bacterial infections of the bronchial tubes and lungs. It is soothing to inflamed mucous membranes and therefore a relief for asthma and croup. It has been applied to ulcers and cancerous growths, sores or other wounds. The oil must not be used internally except in small doses.

EYEBRIGHT: *Euphrasia officinalis*. Also Birdseye, Bright eye. As the name indicates this herb has been used largely for eye disorders and weakness of the eyes. Combined with golden seal it may be prepared as a lotion to soothe inflammation of the eyes and general eye irritation. It has also been applied externally to arrest hemorrhages. It is both a tonic and an astringent.

FENNEL: *Foeniculum officinale*. Also Hinojo. The licorice flavor of this herb makes it a popular seasoning. It has also been used for gas, acid stomach, gout and colic in infants. Reportedly, a tea of the herb is a soothing eyewash, and is used for snake and insect bites. Boiled with barley it seems to increase milk in nursing mothers. It has been known to increase menstrual flow.

FENUGREEK: *Trigonella foenum graecum*. For a sore throat the tea has been said to be an excellent gargle and reportedly, when applied externally to sores it prevents blood poisoning. It has been used to lubricate the intestines and has had a cooling effect on the bowels.

FEVERFEW: *Chrysanthemum parthenium*. Also Featherfew, Featherfoil. This unpleasant tasting herb has been given for hysteria, to promote menstruation and to expel worms.

FIG: *Ficus carica.* A tea has been used to relieve earache, to wash sores and remove soreness and discoloration of bruises and aid in circulation. The milk which escapes when an unripe fruit is broken from a branch has been said to remove warts. The fruit itself is a mild laxative. It has also been used to hasten the healing of boils when split and applied directly, and fig juice, with lemon juice added, is reputed as excellent for coughs and lung diseases.

FIGWORT: *Scrophularia nodosa.* Sometimes called Carpenter's Square, Rosenoble, Scrofula Plant, Throatwort. As a poultice applied directly to wounds, abscesses and skin eruptions, this herb reportedly is a pain reliever and has a cleansing effect. Taken internally as a tea it has been used as a diuretic.

FIREWEED: *Eretchthites hieracifolia.* Common names are Pilewort, Various Leaved Fleabane. The oil of this herb is an astringent and a reported pain reliever, used for hemorrhoids. Being an antispasmodic, it has also been used for colic and hiccoughs. It has also been applied locally for gout and rheumatism.

FIGROOT: *Monotropa uniflora.* Bird's Nest, Convulsion or Fit Weed, Corpse Plant, Dutchman's Pipe, Ice Plant, Indian Pipe, Nest Root, Ova Ova. This sedative and nervine has been used as a replacement for opium and quinine. It has been taken for fevers and spasmodic afflictions, as well as restlessness and nervous irritability.

As a tea with fennel seed it has been used as a douche for inflammation of the uterus and vagina and a wash for irritated eyes.

FLAXSEED: *Linum usitatissium.* Commonly called Linseed or Winterlien. Mixed with other herbs and boiling water, the ground flax seed has been made into a poultice for sores, carbuncles, boils, tumors and inflamed areas. The oil has been helpful for coughs, asthma and pleurisy.

FLEABANE: *Erigeron canadense.* Also Blood Staunch, Butterweed, Colt's, Cow's or Mare's Tail, Fire Weed, and Scabious. Reportedly used as an enema for cholera, dysentery and colon trouble in combination with other herbs. Taken internally it has been used to aid in bladder troubles, scalding urine and hemorrhages from the bowels and uterus.

FLUELLIN: *Linaria elatine.* This is an astringent which has been used both internally and externally. It reportedly stops nosebleed and excessive menstrual bleeding.

FO-TI TIENG: Also known as Hydrocotyle Asiatic. This herb is said to promote clear thinking and rejuvenating effects on brain cells, endocrine and ductless glands. It has been used also for treatment of fevers and piles.

FRINGE TREE: *Chionanthus virginica.* Sometimes known as Old Man's Beard, Snowdrop Tree. Applied both as a lotion and an injection, it has been used for digestive complaints as an alterative, diuretic, hepatic and tonic. With other herbs it has been used for gallstones and female disorders.

FUMITORY: *Fumaria officinalis.* Also called Earth Smoke. This is a mild tonic which has been used as a gentle laxative (aperient) and a diuretic. It has also been applied for skin blemishes.

GARLIC: *Allium sativum.* Mixed with honey, a teaspoon of garlic juice has been helpful in cough, colds and asthma. It also increases perspiration, serves as a diuretic and has helped remove mucus from the throat and lungs.

GIANT SOLOMON SEAL: *Convallatia multiflora.* Commonly called Dropberry, Seal Root, Sealwort. Taken internally or applied as a poultice it has been known to be useful for inflammation of the skin or mucous membrane erysipelas), female disorders, neuralgia, to ease pain and disperse congealed blood from blows and bruises. It has also alleviated vomiting.

GELSEMIUM: *Gelsemium nitidum, Gelsemium sempervirens.* Also Wild Woodbine, Yellow Jasmine. This herb is a sedative, nervine and has been used in cases of insomnia. It reportedly relaxes the nervous system, particularly nerves in the arterial blood vessels, relieves neuralgia, toothache, and diarrhea or dysentery resulting from inflamed bowels. It is also a febrifuge and diaphoretic.

GENTIAN: *Gentiana lutea.* Also Baldmoney, Bitter Root, Bitterwort, Felwort. The root of this plant is the most popular of all herbal tonics and stomachics. It has been used to tone the stomach nerves and as a blood purifier. Acting on the liver and spleen, it reportedly is effective for jaundice, improves the appetite, allays dysentery and dyspepsia, and improves digestion. It has been used to improve the appetite, increase circulation and generally invigorate the system. It acts as an emmenagogue and diuretic and is said to act as a counter-poison for insect, snake and animal bites.

GINGER: *Zingiber officinale.* Also African Ginger, Black Ginger, Race Ginger. This popular condiment stimulates the salivary glands and has been used for paralysis of the tongue and sore throat. Taken hot it assists to bring on suppressed menstruation and causes increased perspiration. It is a carminative when combined with other laxative herbs and therefore also used for bronchitis, cholera, gout and nausea. The tea has been used for colds, grippe, and nausea.

GINGER, WILD: *Asarum canadense.* Sometimes called Canadian Snakeroot. Reportedly, taken hot, this herb is a stimulant for use in colds and amenorrhea and acts on the uterus to bring about labor and childbirth and when taken warm it acts as a carminative for digestive and intestinal pains.

GINSENG: *Panax quinquefolia.* Also Five Finger Root, Garantogen, Ninsin, Red Berry. The Chinese have used ginseng for centuries as a preventive and treatment of diseases of all kinds. It also is a diaphoretic when taken hot. It has been used for lung afflictions and for relief of inflammation in the urinary tract. Because it is said to give comfort for headache and backache, it has been used in cases of lumbago, sciatica and rheumatism. It has also been said to increase appetite, allay hiccoughs, and alleviate some problems of eyesight such as double-vision.

GOA: *Andira araroba.* Common names are Araroba, Bahia Powder, Brazil Powder, Chrysarobine, Ringworm Powder. An ointment of the powder has been helpful when applied locally for eczema, acne, psoriasis and other skin diseases. Taken internally, it is said to destroy tapeworm.

GOAT'S RUE: *Galega officinalis.* This herb has been used as a diuretic, to increase the flow and secretion of urine, and a vermifuge to expel worms. It also seems to help promote the flow of milk in nursing mothers.

GOLDEN ROD, SWEET: *Solidago odora.* The fresh or dried leaves make a tea (with peppermint.) The American Indians used this common herb for sore throat and general pain. It has been used also as a diaphoretic for coughs, colds, and for relief of rheumatism.

GOLDEN SEAL: *Hydrastis canadensis*. Also Eye
Balm, Eye Root, Ground Raspberry, Indian
Plant, Jaundice Root, Ohio Curcuma, Orange
Root, Turmeric Root, Yellow Eye, Yellow Indian Paint, Yellow Paint Root, Yellow Puccoon.
This herb is one of the best and most generally
effective remedies of all. It is used widely in conjunction with other herbs and is useful alone. It
reportedly has a good effect on all mucous membranes and body tissues; it is excellent for all
catarrhal conditions, whether of the throat,
nose, bronchial passages, intestines, stomach or
bladder, is a tonic for spinal nerves and helpful
in spinal meningitis. It has also been combined
with hops and skullcap for this purpose. It has
been said to alleviate pyorrhea or sore gums by
brushing the teeth and gums with the tea. The
tea has also been used as an eyewash and for
sores and skin diseases such as eczema, ringworm and smallpox. For throat troubles, such as
tonsilitis, it has been combined with a little
myrrh and cayenne. This same combination reportedly improves the appetite and aids digestion. It has been used to equalize the circulation
and, combined with skullcap and red pepper,
strengthen the heart. For ulcers of the stomach
and duodenum, for dyspepsia and enlarged tonsils or mouth sores, it has been used with myrrh.
Taken frequently in small doses it is said to alleviate nausea during pregnancy. As a snuff it reportedly helps nose problems. It has also been
used to treat bowel and bladder disorders (with
alum) and as a laxative. This has also been used

for treating hemorrhoids and prostate problems. The herb in tincture form or taken internally has been used for leucorrhea and ulcers of the vagina and uterus.

GOOSEBERRY: *Ribes oxyacanthoides.* Also Feverberry, Groser. Besides its popular use as a fruit in cooking and preserves, a warm tea has been taken to reduce fever and colds. The wine has been taken as a tonic.

GRAPE, WILD: *Vitis.* The wine made from grapes has been taken as a tonic appetizer to increase and improve digestion. It reportedly will reduce acid conditions of the urine and is slightly laxative and diuretic.

GOTU-KOLA: This is said to be a longevity herb and is known for its revitalizing effects on the brain and body. It also acts as a diuretic which stimulates kidney and bladder.

GRAVEL ROOT: *Eupatorium purpureum.* The root of this plant is used as a diuretic and stimulant.

GRINDELLA: *Grindelia camporum.* Sometimes referred to as Gum Plant. This is often combined with euphorbia and Yerba Santa for asthma and bronchitis. It has also been used as a tonic and diuretic.

GROUND IVY: *Glechoma hederacea.* Synonyms are Alehoof, Gill-go-over-the-ground, Haymaids, and Runaway Jack. As an astringent it reportedly works well as a poultice, in combination with camomile or yarrow, applied to abscesses. As a diuretic it has been used for kidney ailments and dyspepsia. It has been used as an antiscorbutic.

GROUNDSEL: *Senecio vulgaris*. This garden weed has been used as a hepatic and a diuretic, and, in stronger doses, as a purgative and emetic.

HARTSTONGUE: *Scolopendrium vulgare*. Has been used as a mild laxative and to relieve coughs. It has also been used as a deobstruent for the liver, spleen and bladder.

HAWTHORN: *Crataegus oxycantha*. Also Haw, May, Whitethorn. This herb should be used under a doctor's direction as a tonic for the heart. It has been found helpful in arteriosclerosis and dyspnea.

HEARTSEASE: *Viola tricolor*. Wild Pansy. This is a diaphoretic and diuretic and has been used as a very mild treatment for skin eruptions.

HEDGE MUSTARD: *Sisymbrium officale*. The dried and powdered herb has been used in connection with hoarseness and weak lungs.

HELLEBORE, FALSE: *Adonis vernalis*. This heart tonic should be used with a doctor's supervision. It has also been helpful in kidney ailments.

HEMP (See Indian hemp)

HENNA LEAVES: *Lawsonia inermis*. Also Alcanna, Egyptian Privet, Jamaican Mignonette. The bark of this plant is known for its use as a dye, while the leaves have been used for jaundice and skin infections (including leprosy), and the root as an astringent.

HOLLYHOCK: *Althaea rosea.* Part of the mallow family, its demulcent and emollient properties are similar to those of the ground and marsh mallow.

HOLY THISTLE: *Carbenia benedicta.* Blessed Thistle, Cardus, Spotted Thistle. Though used mainly for digestive problems, this tonic and diaphoretic has reportedly proven helpful in curing colds and to promote the secretion of milk. There are also claims for its reducing headaches and migraines and purifying the blood. It may be combined with the roots of red dock, yellow dock and burdock.

HONEYSUCKLE: *Lonicera caprifolium.* It facilitates expulsion of mucus from the mucous membrane and it has therefore been used in asthma and disorders of the respiratory organs. It is also a mild laxative and aids in ailments of the liver and spleen.

HOPS: *Humulus lupulus.* A nervine, it is an old-fashioned remedy for insomnia. A pillow stuffed with hops is also said to be effective in bringing on sleep. Hop poultices are reportedly soothing for inflammations, swellings, boils, tumors and old ulcers. It is an anodyne and has been used for earache, toothache, neuralgia, and used for gonorrhea, as a diuretic and a cholagogue. It also has a sedative effect.

HOREHOUND: *Marrubium vulgare.* Hoarhound, Marrubium. Its usefulness as an expectorant has been declaimed for hundreds of years and it is probably one of the best known herbal remedies for coughs, croup, colds, hoarseness, and pulmonary ailments. When taken hot it acts as a diaphoretic, producing profuse perspiration. The syrup has also been taken for asthma and difficult breathing. Taken warm, the tea is reportedly a mild laxative and brings on retarded menstruation. It has also been used to eliminate poisons and expel afterbirth. It has been used externally for skin diseases and to cleanse sores and ulcers. It is this herb from which the popular candy is made.

HOREHOUND, BLACK: *Ballota nigra.* Also Crantz, Marrubium Nigrum. This is similar to white horehound (*Marrubium vulgare,* above) in its diaphoretic, expectorant, and stimulant qualities, and is used similarly.

HORSEMINT: *Monarda punctata.* This has been used in skin diseases such as athlete's foot, impetigo, psoriasis and ringworm. It is also an antiseptic, and a stimulant and nervine. It has been known to expel wind from the bowels and increase the flow of urine. It also acts as a diaphoretic, causing perspiration.

HORSERADISH: *Cochlearia armoracia.* This is now mainly used as a digestive. Modern herbalists rarely prescribe it for dropsy, though its stimulant and diuretic properties are said to be helpful.

HOUSELEEK: *Sempervivum tectorum.* A poultice of the fresh leaves, bruised and applied locally, is said to relieve burns, stings, warts and corns, and reduce discharge, while acting as an astringent.

HYDRANGEA: *Hydrangea aborescens.* Also Sevenbarks. Reportedly used for bladder and kidney troubles, rheumatism, paralysis, scurvy and dropsy. It also acts as a sialagogue.

HYSSOP: *Hyssopus officinalis.* This is a customary ingredient in cough and cold prescriptions and for other pulmonary conditions and asthma. It is a cleanser and, taken with honey, it reportedly destroys intestinal worms. With figs it is said to cleanse the intestines and reduce secretion of lymphatic fluid from body cavities or tissues. It has also helped restore the spleen to normal when taken with figs. Boiled with wine and applied directly to a bruise, it has been known to remove the discoloration. The green herb may be sprinkled on a cut or wound to speed healing.

ICELAND MOSS: *Cetraria islandica.* Also called Iceland Lichen. Besides its considerable nutritive value, the demulcent quality of this lichen affects the lungs, reportedly relieving obstinate coughs, bronchial catarrh and other pulmonary complaints.

INDIAN HEMP: *Pilocorpus selloanus.* Sometimes called Brazilian Jaborandi Root. The tea has been used to stimulate growth of the hair by massaging it into the scalp. It has been taken internally for mumps, or applied as a poultice to reduce the swelling. Its action as an expectorant makes it helpful in breaking up colds and influenza. It has been said to be effective in various fevers, in diabetes, dropsy, jaundice, pleurisy. It is a diaphoretic and causes profuse perspiration.

IPECAC: *Psychotria Ipecacuanha, Cephaelis.* A mouthwash and gargle for pyorrhea has been reported to be soothing. It has been used for coughs and colds, since it is an expectorant and diaphoretic. Taken internally in small doses it has been known to relieve dysentery. Larger doses may cause vomiting.

JAMBUL: *Eugenia jambolana.* Common names are Java Plum, Jamun. It is claimed that the seeds of this plant are able to reduce blood sugar to an extent great enough to be a treatment for diabetes mellitus.

JEWEL WEED: *Impatiens aurea.* Also called Balsam Weed, Pale or Spotted Touch-me-not, Speckled Jewels. It has been said that the juice of the plant may be applied directly to remove corns, warts, and other skin growths and that it also relieves ringworm.

JUNIPER BERRY: *Juniperus communis.* Also Horse

Savin Berries. As a diuretic, the berries and bark are helpful in bladder, kidney and urinary problems. It has been combined with other herbs as a douche for leucorrhea, and to treat gonorrhea, dropsy and scorbutic diseases. Other herbs used in combination with juniper are broom, buchu, cleavers, and uvu ursi. As a spray the berries are excellent for fumigation and they have been chewed or gargled as a disinfectant. Bathing the skin with a juniper solution is said to be beneficial for itches, scabs and even leprosy. Drinking the infusion is reported to help hemorrhoids and prostate troubles, aid in digestion and rid the bowels of worms. Too large a dose may cause irritation of the urinary passages.

JURUBEBA: *Solanum insidiosum.* An emmenagogue, it has been used for liver and spleen disorders.

KELP: *Fucus vesiculosis.* Common names are Black Tany, Bladderwrack, Bladder Fucus, Sea Oak, Seawrack, and Seaweed. Because of its high content of iodine, kelp is especially beneficial to the thyroid and therefore valuable for obesity. Other minerals in this plant are manganese, silicon, calcium, sulphur, copper and iron. These are reported to be effective in toning the skin, to prevent falling hair, strengthen fingernails, prevent indigestion, relieve anemia, and strengthen tissues in the brain and heart. It has also been used to cleanse toxic substances from the colon and thereby relieve nervous disorders, headaches and kidney troubles caused by the presence of these poisons.

KNAPWEED: *Centaurea nigra.* Also Black Ray Thistle, Hardhead, Ironweed, Star Thistle. This herb has been used like gentian as a general tonic and is said to be equally effective.

LADIES' MANTLE: *Alchemilla vulgaris,* or Lion's Foot. As an astringent and nervine it has been used for excessive menstruation, and also used for spasmodic nervous problems.

LADIES' SLIPPER: *Cyprepedium pubescens.* Sometimes called American Valerian, Moccasin Flower, Nerveroot, Noah's Ark. The rhizome of this flowering plant is an antispasmodic, nervine and tonic, and therefore helpful in nervous diseases and hysteria. It is said to relieve pain and has no narcotic effect.

LARKSPUR: *Delphinium consolida.* Sometimes called Lark's Claw or Heel, Knight's Spur. A tincture of this herb has been used for external parasites and insects, such as hair lice. Taken in small doses it has also been used in the relief of asthma and dropsy.

LAVENDER: *Lavandula vera.* A tea made by steeping the flowers is said to be a good general tonic and has been used to allay nausea and prevent fainting. It is also an aromatic. The flowers and leaves are most commonly used for their fragrant scent.

LEMON: *Citrus limonum.* A refreshing drink, lemon juice has been used as a tonic and cold remedy. It has been helpful in fevers, headache, and other cold symptoms, especially coughs.

LICORICE: *Glycirrhiza glabra.* This popular ingredient in candy has been used as an expectorant, to soothe irritation, and promote bowel action.

LILY OF THE VALLEY: *Convallaria majalis.* Also May lily. The root has been used for calming the heart. Reportedly helpful in convulsions of all types, and is said to generally clear and strengthen the brain and alleviate dizziness.

LINDEN (or LIME FLOWERS) : *Tilia europoea, Tilia americana.* The flowers of this tree are both nervine and stimulant. They are a popularly used remedy to help clear up excess flow of mucus from inflamed mucous membranes of the nose and throat. They reportedly have an excellent effect on the digestive and nervous system. The tea has long been substituted for the more widely used English and Chinese teas.

LOBELIA: *Lobelia inflata.* Also called Asthma Weed, Emetic Herb, Eyebright, Gag Root, Indian Tobacco, Puke Weed, Vomit Wort. There is a great deal of controversy over this herb. While many herbalists contend that it is the most valuable botanic remedy, it is classified in some countries as a poison. It is used chiefly as an emetic and an expectorant, for fevers, pneumonia, meningitis, pleurisy, etc. It has been applied as an enema with catnip; with pleurisy root for pleurisy; with slippery elm bark for poultices to treat abscesses, boils and carbuncles. It is also reported to be a powerful relaxant and helpful in asthma and spasmodic vomiting.

LOW MALLOW: *Malva rotundifolia.* Also Cheese Plant, Dwarf Mallow. This has both a demulcent and emollient action and has been used to soothe inflammation and irritation of alimentary, respiratory, and urinary organs.

LUCERNE: *Medicago sativa.* Commonly called Alfalfa. Used as a tea or powdered and mixed with cider vinegar and honey, it is reportedly used for arthritis and to aid in weight gain. It seems to be a strength-giving tonic as well.

LUNGWORT: *Pulmonaria officinalis.* Also called Jerusalem cowslip, Jerusalem sage, spotted comfrey. Because of its action as a demulcent, an expectorant, a pectoral and a mucilaginous, lungwort is used for colds, coughs, influenza, and for diseases of the chest and lungs. It decreases excessive menstruation and has been used as a bath for genital ulcers.

LYCOPODIUM: *Lycopodium clavatum.* Sometimes called Common Club Moss, Foxtail, Lamb's Tail, Vegetable Sulphur, Wolf's Claws. The spores of this plant have been used as a medicinal dusting powder. Taken internally it is reported helpful for indigestion and diseases of the lungs and kidneys. Because of its reported healing effects on mucous membranes, it has been used for swellings of arteries and to relieve itching of the anus.

MAGNOLIA: *Magnolia glauca.* Common names are Bay Beaver Tree, Holly Bay, Indian Bark, Red Bay, Red Laurel, Swamp Laurel, Swamp Sassafras, Sweet Magnolia. There are claims that the bark of the magnolia tree reduces craving for tobacco. It has been used as a tonic and is reportedly helpful in intermittent fever, dysentery, dyspepsia, and erysipelas. For leucorrhea it has been used in a douche. Externally it has been applied directly for skin diseases.

MANDRAKE: *Podophyllum peltatum.* Also called American Mandrake, Duck's Foot, Ground Lemon, Hog Apple, Indian Apple, May Apple, Raccoon Berry, Wild Lemon, Yellow Berry. The rhizome of this plant is a hepatic and purgative, but it is so powerful that it should only be taken under the direction of a physician. It has often been combined with other herbs to regulate liver and bowels, for uterine disorders and intermittent fever.

MAPLE, RED: *Acer rubrum,* or Swamp Maple. This is a popular salve, used originally by the American Indians, for sore eyes. It is also an astringent and reportedly helps eliminate fluid discharges.

MARIGOLD; *Calendula officinalis.* The flowers and leaves have been made into a salve for direct application to skin eruptions, as in measles, and

to varicose veins and chronic ulcers. A hot fermentation is said to relieve sore muscles. It has
also been taken for amenorrhea.

MARJORAM: *Origanum-marjorana*. Also Sweet
Marjoram, Knotted Marjoram. This herb is often used with gentian and camomile and is reportedly an excellent general tonic. It has been
helpful for indigestion, sour stomach, nausea,
colic, loss of appetite, and suppressed menstruation. For toothache a few drops of oil on the
aching tooth is said to stop the pain. It is also a
diaphoretic when taken hot and is therefore
able to cleanse the system and expel poisons
from the body.

MARSH MALLOW: *Althaea officinalis*. Sometimes
called Althaea, Guimauve, Mallards, Mortifica-
tion Root, Schloss Tea, Sweet Weed, Wymote.
This herb is said to be very soothing and healing and taken both internally and externally.
It has been used as a poultice for sore or inflamed parts, as a tea to bathe sore eyes, and as a
douche for irritation of the vagina. It is also a
mucilaginous and has been taken for lung troubles, hoarseness, catarrh and pneumonia. As a
diuretic it has been helpful in kidney diseases.

MASTERWORT: *Heracleum lanatum*. Sometimes
known as Cow Parsnip, Madnep, Madness,
Youthwort. This plant is reportedly a good antispasmodic for asthma and epilepsy. As a carminative it has caused gases to be expelled from
the gastrointestinal tract. It has been taken for

colds, kidney stones, suppressed or painful menstruation, cramps, dropsy, palsy and apoplexy. Externally it is said to be a good wash for sores and ulcers.

MEADOWSWEET: *Spiraea ulmaria.* Common names are Bridewort, Dolloft, Queen of the Meadow. This herb is mild and therefore reported safely used for infantile diarrhea. It also has aromatic, tonic and diuretic qualities which make it popular for use in herb beers.

MELILOT: *Melilotus officinalis.* Also King's Clover. An infusion can be made for flatulence. It is also an emollient used in poultices. See also White Clover.

MESCAL BUTTONS: *Lopophora lewinii, Anhalonium lewinii.* Also called Pellote. Very small amounts of the tea have been taken to relieve angina pectoris, but an excessive amount may cause vomiting. It is also a narcotic and can bring on a stupor or complete unconsciousness.

MILKWEED: *Asclepias syriaca.* Sometimes called Silkweed, Silky Swallow Wort. This is reportedly an excellent remedy for gallstones when used with marsh mallow. It is a diuretic and therefore has been used in dropsy and kidney and bowel troubles. It has also been taken for asthma, stomach complaints, female disorders and scrofulous conditions of the blood.

MINT: *Monarda punctata.* Also Horsemint, Origanum. A carminative, the tea has reportedly caused expulsion of gas from the stomach and intestines. It is also an emmenagogue and has been known to bring on suppressed menstruation. It is very quieting and reportedly eases pain. It is also a stimulant and diuretic, has been used to increase the flow of urine and for nausea and vomiting.

MISTLETOE: *Viscum flavescens.* Also Bird Lime, Golden Bough. As an antispasmodic and nervine the leaves of this plant have been used for epilepsy, convulsions, and hysteria. It reportedly acts as a tonic and is recommended for suppressed and painful menstruation, uterine hemorrhages, and has been suggested for high blood pressure. It is also a narcotic, producing sleep, stupor, or unconsciousness.

MOTHERWORT: *Leonurus cardiaca.* Also Lion's Ear, Lion's Tail, Throwwort. This plant is an emmenagogue, reportedly increasing menstrual flow; a nervine and an antispasmodic, said to relieve menstrual cramps. It has also been helpful in nervous complaints, convulsions, hysteria, and liver affections. Reportedly it will kill worms and is a good remedy for chest colds.

MOUNTAIN FLAX: *Linum cartharticum.* Also known as Purging Flax. This herb is a laxative and cathartic and rarely causes griping. It has been used with diuretics for bladder and gallstones and dropsy. Sometimes it is taken with gentian and calumba root.

MOUSEAR: *Hieracium pilosella.* Common names

are Hawkweed, and Pilosella. As an astringent
and expectorant this reportedly makes a useful
medicine for whooping cough and other
coughs.

MUGWORT: *Artemisia vulgaris.* Sometimes called
Felon Herb. This is an emmenagogue. It is said
to have been helpful for fevers, gout, kidney
and bladder stones and swellings. A drink of the
warm infusion has often relieved bowel or stomach pain.

MULLEIN: *Verbascum thapsus.* Also called Bul-
lock, Candle Flower, Cow's Lungwort, Flannel
Flower, Hare's Beard, Lungwort, Pig Taper,
Shepherd's Club, Velvet Plant, Verbascum
Flower, Woolen Blanket Herb. The leaves and
root of this plant are used internally and externally in many ways. As a poultice the herb has
been known to relieve swelling of all types. A
fermentation has been used for piles, tumors,
mumps, tonsilitis, and sore throats. It has been
taken internally for dysentery, diarrhea, bleeding bowels, dropsy, catarrh, swollen joints. A
tea from the leaves has been taken for asthma,
all lung afflictions, and hay fever. It is also reportedly good as a gargle, for toothache and
for cleansing open sores. A tea made from the
flowers is said to induce sleep, relieve pain, and
in large doses act as a physic. Inhalations of
fumes from the burning root have been used
for treating asthma.

MUIRA-PUAMA: *Liriosma ovata.* The powdered

root of this herb has been used as a nerve stimulant.

MUSTARD: *Sinapis alba*. Also known as kedlock. A laxative, stimulant, condiment and emetic. A mustard plaster made with this herb has been used to relieve irritation of the kidney. Reportedly used to induce vomiting.

MYRRH: *Balsamodendron myrrh*. Also known as Gum Myrrh Tree. An antiseptic, this reportedly is an effective treatment for pyorrhea and also removes halitosis. As an ointment combined with golden seal it is said to be an excellent injection for piles. With charcoal it has been used to hasten healing of sores and ulcers. As an expectorant it has been taken for cough, asthma, tuberculosis and all other chest afflictions. It is both a tonic and stimulant and has been used for bronchial and lung diseases. As a stimulant, it has been used in cases of shock and prostration.

NETTLE: *Urtica dioica*. Also known as Stinging Nettle. The tea made from the root and leaves of the nettle is said to be an excellent hair tonic, bringing back natural-color and removing dandruff. It has also been given for dropsy, kidney troubles and bladder stones, when a diuretic is needed. The boiled leaves are a styptic but must be used carefully as they may cause blistering if left in contact with the skin too long. It has also been taken internally for hemorrhaging, and as an expectorant and emmenagogue. For chronic rheumatism the bruised leaves have been rubbed on the skin. With Seawrack it has been used as a reducing aid. The green leaves, cooked like spinach, are said to be a good blood purifier.

NIGHT-BLOOMING CEREUS: *Cereus grandiflorus.* Also Sweet-scented Cactus. As a heart stimulant this herb is reportedly able to bring relief in angina pectoris, palpitations, cardiac neuralgia and irritations of the prostate gland, bladder and kidneys. It has also been used for headaches during menstruation and acts as a diuretic.

NUTMEG: *Nigella sativa.* Common names are Bishop's Wort, Black Caraway, Black Cumin, Flower Seed, Nigella Seed, Small Fennel Flower. This popular seasoning is a sialagogue, increasing the flow of saliva, and stimulating the appetite. It has been known to prevent gas from forming in the bowels, intestines or stomach, and reportedly brings on or increases menstruation. It is a deobstruent and diaphoretic.

NUX VOMICA: *Strychnos nux vomica.* Also Poison Nut, Quaker Buttons. The seeds of this herb have been used as a general tonic and stimulant and are reportedly valuable for impotence, general debility and neuralgia. It stimulates peristalsis and has thus been used as an aid for constipation. An excessive dose could be poisonous.

OATS: *Avena sativa.* Sometimes called Groats, Panicle Oats, White Oats. A drink of oatmeal has been taken for indigestion and constipation and as a general tonic. A poultice of oatmeal has been applied to relieve itching. It has also been used as a nerve tonic and seems to strengthen cardiac muscles. Because of its reported relaxing effect on the nerves, oatmeal may facilitate sleep in cases of insomnia. It is also reported to remove spots on the skin and freckles when applied as a mash.

OLIVE: *Olea europae.* Also Lucca Oil, Provence Oil, Salad Oil, Sweet Oil, Virgin Oil. This has been used for constipation, often being substituted for castor oil. It is also reportedly used for intestinal worms and to remove stony deposits from the bile. Externally it has been applied directly to burns, scalds, bruises and other skin conditions. It is also reported helpful for rheumatism.

ONION: *Allium cepa.* Boiled onion has been eaten to relieve colds and to stimulate the kidneys. Roasted and made into a poultice it has been applied to tumors or ulcers and reportedly will help draw out pus. The same poultice has been said to be helpful for earaches.

ORIGANUM: *Origanum vulgare.* Also Mountain Mint, Wild Marjoram, Winter Marjoram, Winter Sweet. This plant reportedly helps toothache, swellings, sprains, boils and sore throat. It has been said that it is strengthening to the stomach and promotes appetite, relieves sour stomach, expels gas, relieves dyspepsia, colic and nausea. It seems to be soothing for bad coughs and consumption. It is also a diuretic, and an emmenagogue.

OX-EYE DAISY: *Chrysanthemum leucanthemum.* Also Field Daisy, Horsegowan, Marguerite, Moon Daisy. This herb has a tonic effect similar to camomile. It has been used in whooping cough and asthma for its antispasmodic properties, and it is reportedly used externally for wounds and ulcers and as a douche for leucorrhea. Large does taken internally have been said to produce vomiting.

PARAGUAY TEA: *Ilex paraguayensis.* Also Brazil Tea, Jesuit's Tea, Mate, Yerba Mate. The leaves of this herb have a diuretic effect and, because of the presence of caffeine, are also a stimulant. It has been used for rheumatism and gout and reportedly, in large doses, acts as a purgative.

PARSLEY: *Petroselinum sativum.* Also called March. The root and leaves of this well known garden plant have been used for liver and kidney problems, including stones or obstructions, dropsy, difficult urination, jaundice and various fevers. It is also reported to have been used for syphilis and gonorrhea. It has also been classed as a preventive herb. It has been used with buchu, black haw and cramp bark for female troubles. Externally a hot fermentation has helped to relieve insect bites and stings. A poultice of the bruised leaves has been applied to swollen glands and swollen breasts, or to dry up milk. The tea will reportedly kill vermin in the hair.

PARSLEY PIERT: *Alchemilla arvensis,* or Breakstone Parsley. An infusion of this herb has been given to regulate bladder and kidney functions.

PASSION FLOWER: *Passiflora incranata.* Sometimes called Maypops, Passion Vine, Wild Passion Flower. As a nervine this herb is reportedly helpful in nervous conditions, such as insomnia, hysteria, high blood pressure, headache, and asthma. In some cases it has relieved neuralgia pains.

PEACH: *Amygdalus persica.* The leaves of this common tree have been used as a sedative, a laxative, or a demulcent. They are said to relieve morning sickness in pregnancy and dyspepsia. They have also been taken for abdominal inflammation and to expel worms. It has been said that for bladder and uterine disorders a tea may be imbibed, and in small doses the hot tea helps reduce vomiting. For sores or wounds, a powder of the bark or leaves has been applied to hasten healing. The buds are said to restore hair growth in baldness.

PELLITORY-OF-THE-WALL: *Parietaria officinalis.* As a diuretic this herb has been used for bladder and kidney disorders, such as gravel or suppressed urine. It is often used with wild carrot and parsley piert.

PENNYROYAL: *Hedeoma pulegioides.* Also Mock Pennyroyal, Squaw Mint, Stinking Balm, Thickweed, Tickweed. As a sudorific this herb has been taken to reduce fevers. It is also an emmenagogue and has been said to bring on suppressed menstruation, and should not be used by a pregnant woman. It is also reportedly used for toothache, gout, leprosy, colds, consumption, congested chest and lungs, jaundice, dropsy, itch, ulcers, to ward off and heal insect bites, and stings; the oil has been used in liniments. As a carminative it has been used to relieve intestinal pain, colic, and griping. Its sedative effect reportedly soothes nervous headache, hysteria and convulsions. Used as a poultice and wash it has been used to relieve bruises and skin diseases.

PEONY: *Paeonia officinalis.* This is reportedly used as a tonic and antispasmodic for chorea and epilepsy.

PEPPERMINT: *Mentha piperita.* Balm Mint, Brandy Mint. This is an old and popular household herb. It is a general stimulant, stronger than liquor, and will reportedly bring back warmth and equilibrium to the body in case of fainting and dizziness. It has been said to strengthen the heart, aid in digestion and soothe indigestion. It has also been used to relieve headaches and is better for the body than drugs taken for the same purpose. The leaves, chewed until they are easily swallowed, are said to have the same effect as the tea. The oil has been applied locally for rheumatism and neuralgia. Peppermint enemas are reported to be excellent in cholera and colon troubles.

PERUVIAN BARK: *Cinchona calisaya.* Also Calisaya Bark, Jacket Bark, Jesuit's Bark, Yellow Bark, Yellow Cinchona. This bark has been taken as quinine but is itself harmless. It is a good febrifuge, and has been used in abating and reducing fevers. It has also been taken for dyspepsia, neuralgia, epilepsy, and female debility. It is said to strengthen the lungs, and has therefore been used for pneumonia.

PERIWINKLE: *Vinca major.* This has been taken as a drink for internal hemorrhages and diarrhea, as a gargle for sore throat, and as a douche for leucorrhea and excessive menstruation. There is some evidence that this herb is beneficial in diabetes.

PILEWORT: *Ranunculus ficaria.* Also Lesser Celandine, Small Celandine. As the name indicates, this has been used for hemorrhoids because of its astringent and detergent properties.

PINKROOT: *Spigelia marilandica.* Sometimes American Wormwort, Carolina Pink, Demerara Pinkroot, Indian Pink, Maryland Pink, Wormgrass. This is one of the best vermifuges and has been taken with a laxative such as senna.

PITCHER PLANT: *Serracenia purpurea.* Also Flytrap, Saddleplant, Watercup. The powder root of this plant has been used to treat smallpox. It is a laxative and diuretic and is reportedly helpful for derangements of the stomach, liver and kidneys.

PLANTAIN: *Plantago major*. Also Cuckoo's Bread, Englishman's Foot, Ribwort, Ripplegrass, Waybread. To check bleeding, the fresh leaves pounded into a paste have been applied and reportedly have a soothing, cooling and healing effect. It has also been applied for skin irritations and diseases as a tea. It has been injected for hemorrhoids or applied externally on a piece of gauze. Reportedly used as a douche for leucorrhea and syphilis and as a tea for diarrhea, kidney and bladder trouble and their accompanying symptoms. The mashed green leaves have also been applied as a poultice for insect and snake bites, boils, carbuncles or tumors. As an astringent, plantain contracts tissues and has been used for excessive flow in menstruation. It has also been used for dropsy, toothache, inflamed eyes, as a vermifuge, and, with yellowdock, as a wash for itching skin, ringworm, or running sores.

PLEURISY ROOT: *Asclepias tuberosa*. Also Butterfly Weed, Canada Root, Flux Root, Orange Swallow Wort, Tuber Root, White Root, Wind Root. As the name suggests it has been used in bronchial and pulmonary diseases, including colds, grippe and pleurisy. It is reportedly good for the kidneys and to treat suppressed menstruation, dysentery, scarlet and rheumatic fevers, typhus, measles and other fevers.

POKE ROOT: *Phytolacca decandra*. Sometimes called American Nightshade, Cuncer Jalap, Garget, Pigeon Berry, Pocan Bush, Red Ink Plant,

Scoke Coakum, Virginia Poke. The leaves of this plant have often been eaten as a vegetable, which acts as a general tonic. It is reportedly good for treating enlarged glands, particularly the thyroid, and therefore used as a treatment for goiter. Taken internally or used as a poultice, it has been applied to growths and chronic enlargement of bones caused by injury. A tea has been used for treating the skin.

PRICKLY ASH: *Xanthoxylum americanum.* Also Suterberry, Toothache Bush. This has been used widely as a stimulant and for general debility as a tonic. It has been effective, reportedly, for paralysis of the tongue and mouth and for rheumatism and hepatitis. The berries are said to be helpful for poor circulation.

PSYLLA: *Plantago psyllium, Plantago ispaghula.* Also Branching Plantain, Flea Seed, Flea Wort. This herb is said to have the effect of removing toxins from the intestines and colon, toning and ridding them of sluggishness. It has been used therefore for colitis, hemorrhoids, and ulcers.

PULSATILLA: *Anemone pulsatilla.* Sometimes called Easter Flower, Meadow Anemone, Passe Flower, Wind Flower. Because of its nervine and antispasmodic qualities this has been taken by women for nervousness and fatigue, especially when it results from menstruation. It is also reported good for all of the mucous membranes.

PURSLANE: *Portulaca oleracea.* Sometimes called Pussley, Portulaca. This is an especially nutri-

tious plant and the leaves may be served un-
cooked and included in salads. It may also be
steamed or cooked and served like spinach. Its
effect is to cool, and it has been taken for fevers
and to stimulate the appetite.

PURPLE LOOSE-STRIFE: *Lythrum salicaria.* Sometimes known as Purple Grass or Willow Strife.
This is most often used with other herbs. It is an
astringent which has been said to be especially
helpful in diarrhea. It has also been used to reduce fevers and as an alterative.

QUASSIA: *Picrasma excelsa.* Also Bitter Wood or
Bitter Ash. Cups known as "bitter cups" are
made of the wood from quassia trees; water allowed to steep in the cup acquires the medicinal properties of the wood. Otherwise chips of
the wood may be soaked in water, which has
been taken in small doses for expelling worms
and as a bitter tonic. It is also said to dispel the
desire for alcohol.

QUEEN OF THE MEADOW: *Eupatorium purpureum.*
Also Gravel Root, Joe Pye, Kidney Root, Purple
Boneset, Trumpet Weed. This herb is reportedly used with blue cohosh, lily root, marsh mallow, and uva ursi for female disorders, diabetes,
and Bright's disease. It has also been taken
alone or with other herbs for urinary and bladder disorders (e.g. stones), dropsy, rheumatism
and neuralgia. It is a mild nervine.

QUEEN'S DELIGHT: *Stillingia sylvatica Linne;* Euphorbiacae. Also Silver Leaf, Queen's Root, Yaw Root. Reportedly used for purifying the blood and for conditions such as scrofula or infectious diseases. It has been said to stimulate action of the kidneys. Combined with sundew it has been taken for laryngitis or as a cough remedy; with bittersweet for eczema and as a relaxant; and with milkweed and Indian tobacco for bronchitis.

QUINCE: *Cydonia oblonga, Pyrus cydonia.* Sometimes known as Cydonium, Cydonia Vulgaris, Semen Cydoniae. The seeds of the quince fruit are sometimes used in a skin and hair lotion; their effect is to contract tissues and skin. For conjunctivitis it is reportedly a soothing eyewash, and it has been taken for diarrhea and dysentery. A lotion of the crushed seeds and water is said to make a healing cream for skin abrasions or cracks in the mucous membrane.

RAGWORT: *Senecio jacobaea.* Also Dog Standard, Fireweed, Ragweed, St. James' Wort, Staggerwort, Stinking Nanny. As a decoction this reportedly makes a good gargle and has been applied externally to ulcers, wounds and inflamed eyes. It is a diaphoretic as well and has been used for coughs, colds, influenza, catarrh, sciatica or rheumatic pains.

RAGWORT: *Senecio aureus.* Cocash Weed, Cough Weed, False Valerian, Golden Senecio, Liferoot, Squaw Weed, Uncum, Waw Weed. Because of its effect on the female organs, it has been used for leucorrhea and amenorrhea. It is said to relieve urinary diseases and gravel.

RASPBERRY: *Rubus stringosus.* A tea of the leaves has been a popular drink during pregnancy, as it is believed to aid in parturition. It is an astringent and has been used as a mouthwash and gargle and for cleansing wounds and ulcers. It has been taken with ginger and pennyroyal for stomach and bowel disorders in children, and with slippery elm as a poultice. It also has been claimed that it decreases menstrual flow.

RED PEPPER: See "Cayenne."

RED ROOT: *Ceanothus Americanus.* Synonyms are Bobea, Jersey Tea, Mountain Sweet, New York Tea, Walpole Tea, Wild Snowball. Because of its astringent and expectorant properties, the root of this plant has been used for dysentery, asthma, bronchitis, whooping cough, consumption, tonsillitis, and piles or hemorrhoids. It is said to be especially effective in any spleen trouble and diabetes.

RHATANY, PERUVIAN: *Krameria triandra.* Also Rhatanhia. As an astringent this herb is reportedly used to stop bleeding or hemorrhaging, in menstrual disorders where fluid discharges occur, and has been used in bowel malfunctions. As a tonic it is said to restore strength and muscle tone and has been taken to regain control of sphincter muscles to control incontinence of urine. For pyorrhea a small amount of the powder has been applied to the gums.

RHUBARB: *Rheum palmatum*. Also Rhizoma Rhei or Chinese or Turkish Rhubarb. This is not the ordinary garden variety of rhubarb but a larger member of the same family. An effective cathartic value for its very mild action, it is also an astringent, contracting tissues and tending to alleviate diarrhea and stomach troubles. It is reportedly a stomach tonic taken to improve digestion and increase appetite.

ROCK ROSE: *Helianthemum canadense*. Also Frost Plant, Frost Weed, Frostwort, Scrofula Plant, Sun Rose. A poultice of the leaves reportedly helps ulcers and tumors and it is said to make an excellent gargle for sore throats and scarletina. Taken internally it has aided in diarrhea, syphilis and gonorrhea.

ROSEMARY: *Rosmarinus officinalis*. Also Garden Rosemary, Romero. This herbal tonic has reportedly been used for many years for colds, colic and nerves—including nervous headaches. It has been used as a mouthwash for sore mouth, gums or throat. It has been used too for female disorders and is said to strengthen the eyes and prevent premature baldness.

RUE: *Ruta graveolens*. Also Country Man's Treacle, Garden Rue, Herb of Grace. This is one of the oldest and most internationally-known medicinal herbs. As a tea it is said to relieve

uterine congestion, and has been used in amenorrhea, painful menstruation and has a tonic
effect on the uterus. It reportedly helps in
stomach troubles, including colic, cramps in
the bowels, and is an antispasmodic taken for
convulsions and hysteria. It is also a vermifuge.
Some herbalists recommend a tea of this plant
to clear the mind and relieve headache pain. A
poultice of rue is said to relieve sciatica, gout
and pain in the joints.

ROSE, WILD: *Rose canina.* Also Dog Rose, Brier
Rose. A tea of the leaves and dried petals of the
wild rose bush are used as a tea substitute and it
is said to be soothing to persons with arthritis or
dyspepsia. It has none of the tannic acid of coffee and tea, nor does it have the effect of stimulating the heart. The petals contain acids which
reportedly help to dissolve gallstones and gravel.
The hips, or fruit, contain sixty times the vitamin C of lemons, as well as natural sugar, and
the puree, powder, and extract have been used
to prevent colds.

SAFFRON: *Carthamus tinctorius.* The flowers and
seed of this plant, besides being a popular condiment, have been used for measles, scarlet fever, and other eruptive skin maladies. Because
it is a sudorific it has been taken for colds and
influenza to produce perspiration. It is also an
emmenagogue, reportedly stimulating and increasing menstrual flow. It is also a carminative
and diuretic.

SAGE: *Salvia officinalis.* Also Garden Sage. This favorite among kitchen herbs is a digestive as well. It has been used for sores and ulcers in the mouth, laryngitis and inflamed throat. The healthful tea is reputedly helpful in cases of dyspepsia and gas in the stomach or bowels. As a vermifuge both adults and children may use it. It is a nervine and said to be soothing to the nerves and delirium from fever. As an astringent, it has been used to halt bleeding as well as to cleanse wounds. Reportedly, for liver and kidney trouble the tea is taken internally, as it is for spermatorrhea; to stop the flow of milk in the breasts, the tea is drunk cold; taken hot it reduces fever by producing free perspiration and strengthening circulation. There are also claims for it as a hair restorer and a dandruff remedy.

SAGE, RED: *Salvia colorata.* Sometimes called Purple-Topped Sage. This has been taken for its healing effect in lung trouble, including bronchitis, asthma, coughs, colds, grippe, sore throat and tonsillitis. For diphtheria a gargle with a strong tea of red sage has been said to have a soothing effect. It is also an emmenagogue, having been used to promote menstruation; as a diuretic, detergent, tonic and astringent it is reportedly beneficial in preventing gas or fermentation in the stomach. It is slightly laxative and has been used as a liver cleanser. Taken in cases of nervousness or nervous headache it is said to act as a nervine and a stimulant. As a healing poultice for inflammations, it has been applied for smallpox and measles and has been taken internally for typhoid and scarlet fever.

ST. JOHN'S WORT: *Hypericum perforatum*. An oil of this plant has been applied to wounds, swellings and ulcers to soothe and heal. It is also an expectorant and has been taken for coughs and colds, and its effect as a diuretic has made it useful in disorders of the urinary system.

SANICLE: *Sanicula europaea*. Also Pool Root. Though there have been claims for this as a remedy for consumption, they are unproven. It is, however, a powerful alterative and an astringent which has been taken in diarrhea and leucorrhea and has been used externally for erysipelas and rashes.

SARSAPARILLA: *Smilax*. Though it was first introduced in the 16th century for syphilis, this claim has long since been disproven. It is, though, an excellent alterative and has been used when a blood purifier is indicated. Reportedly an excellent demulcent it has been applied to skin diseases, rheumatism, scrofula and gout. It has been used as an anti-toxin, an eyewash, a diuretic, and a carminative.

SASSAFRAS: *Sassafras officinale*. Sometimes referred to as Ague Tree, Cinnamon Wood, Kuntze Saloip, Saxifrax. This is a favorite spring tonic reportedly taken to purify the blood and cleanse the entire system. It has been said to relieve colic and gas in the stomach and bowels; that for sore and inflamed eyes it is a soothing bath; and that the oil will relieve a toothache. It has also been applied to skin sores and diseases; claims are made for it as a cure for varicose veins too. Because of its agreeable flavor it may be used to flavor other medicines, and rubbed over the skin it reportedly repels flies.

SAW PALMETTO: *Seronoa serrulata, Sabal serrulata.* Sometimes called Dwarf Palmetto, Pan Palm. This is reportedly a valuable treatment for any disease in which there is excessive discharge of mucus from the head or nose, such as asthma, colds, bronchitis, grippe, whooping cough, and sore throat caused by the mucus. It has been said to be an excellent herb for toning and strengthening glandular tissues and muscles, and has been used, therefore, for debility caused by tuberculosis, or other enfeebling diseases. It has also been used for diseases of the reproductive organs, nephritis, and diabetes.

SCOPOLIS: *Scopola carniolica* or *Scopolia atropoides.* Reportedly, a small amount of this herb acts as a sedative and brings relief from pain and coughs.

SKULLCAP: *Scutellaria lateriflora.* In some areas this is known as Blue Pimpernel, Helmet Flower, Hoodwort, Hooded Willow Herb, Mad Dogweed or Madweed. Combined with other herbs or by itself this has been used as a tonic for the nerves. It acts as an antispasmodic, as well as a pain reliever, and has been taken for neuralgia, delirium tremens, rheumatism, poisonous insect or snake bite, St. Vitus' dance, rabies, fits or convulsions, and epilepsy. With golden seal and cayenne it is reportedly a good heart tonic. The herb deteriorates rapidly from age and heat and should be stored in an airtight container.

SCURVYGRASS: *Cochlearia officinalis.* Also known as Spoonwort. This herb is rarely used now, but before dietetic remedies for scurvy were known, it was recognized as a powerful antiscorbutic.

SEA LAVENDER: *Statice limonium.* Sometimes referred to as Marsh Rosemary. This herb which, in spite of its name, has no scent, is an astringent and has been used as a mouthwash and gargle for inflammation. It has been taken too for some cases in which there are urinary, uterine and vaginal discharges.

SEAWRACK: *Fucus versiculosus.* Also Black Tany, Kelpware, Sea Oak, Bladder Fucus, Bladderwrack. This is an herb reportedly taken for glandular problems, such as goiter, and for obesity. It has been said to have a favorable effect on the kidneys.

SELF-HEAL: *Prunella vulgaris.* Also called All-Heal. As an astringent this has been taken in small doses for internal bleeding, as a douche for leucorrhea, and as a gargle for sore throats.

SENNA: *Cassia acutifolia.* Also known as Locust Plant. Reportedly taken for minor ailments such as dyspepsia and constipation, this is a mild laxative. It should be combined with an aromatic herb (such as ginger) to prevent griping. It has been said to be effective for expelling worms in combination with other herbs.

SHEPHERD'S PURSE: *Capsella bursa pastoris.* Common names are Cocowort, Mother's Heart, Pepper Grass, Pickpocket, Poor Man's Pharmacetty, St. Anthony's Fire, St. James' Weed. This reportedly is used for halting internal hemorrhages of all kinds and to check menstruation; is taken for bleeding piles and hemorrhoids; in intermittent fever; and as a remedy for diarrhea. An infusion has been used for kidney complaints and dropsy. It is sometimes used with pellitory-of-the-wall and juniper berries: Added to coleslaw, it has a delicious peppery flavor.

SIMARUBA: *Simaruba officinalis.* Also Mountain Damson. This herb has been used for aiding digestion and has been taken for loss of appetite, especially during convalescence. It reportedly serves to strengthen the muscles and tone the tissues.

SKUNK CABBAGE: *Ictodes foetidus.* Sometimes called Collard, Fedit Hellebore, Meadow Cabbage, Polecat Weed, Skunk Weed, Swamp Cabbage. This is an old-fashioned remedy for bronchial and lung problems, including tuberculosis, catarrh, asthma, whooping cough, pulmonary consumption, and pleurisy. Externally it has been applied to tumors and sores for relief of pain. It has also been taken for rheumatism, dysentery, nervousness, spasms, convulsions, hysteria, dropsy and epilepsy. It has been used during pregnancy as a general tonic.

SLIPPERY ELM: *Ulmus fulva*. Also Moose Elm, Red Elm. The powdered bark of this tree reportedly makes one of the best poultices for skin eruptions such as boils; it has been said to be healing and soothing and to draw out impurities. Its emollient effect has been used for inflammation of the mucous membranes of the bowels, kidneys and stomach. The tea has been used as an enema and as a douche for inflammation of the vagina. As a nutritious gruel it has been used for general debility and both bronchitis and gastritis reportedly are helped by its soothing and healing properties.

SNAKE ROOT: *Aristolochia serpentaria, Aristolochia reticulata*. A febrifuge that has been taken for typhoid, this herb is also a diaphoretic inducing perspiration, and a stimulant which promotes the activity of the glands. As a tonic it reportedly strengthens the muscles and the tissues. It has also been said to be a pain reliever and antispasmodic.

SOAP TREE: *Quillaja saponaria*. Common names are Panama Bark, Quillaia, Soap bark. Reportedly for coughs or bronchial and lung ailments, this herb has also been applied externally to cleanse skin eruptions. It is also a diuretic.

SOLOMON'S SEAL: *Convallaria polygonatum.* Reportedly, solomon's seal is prepared as a poultice for inflammations and wounds and a wash to soothe erysipelas, poison ivy, and other sores. As a tea it has been taken internally for female disorders and neuralgia.

SORREL: *Rumex acetosa.* Also Garden Sorrel, Sourgrass. Sorrel has been taken as a blood cleanser and for its warming effect on the heart. It is a vermifuge too. It has been said to reduce excessive menstruation and stomach hemorrhage. Reportedly, a tea from the flowers has been used for gravel in the kidneys, black jaundice, internal ulcers, scrofula, and for skin diseases. The leaves, eaten like spinach, are very nutritious.

SOUTHERN WOOD: *Artemisia abrotanum.* Common names are Lad's Love, Old Man. A garden plant cultivated for its pleasant aroma, reportedly taken to remove menstrual obstruction, combined with mugwort and pennyroyal. The fragrance is claimed to be a repellent of various insects, especially moths.

SPEARMINT: *Mentha viridis.* Also called Mint. As a diuretic and carminative, spearmint has been used for gas in the stomach and bowels, colic, dyspepsia, nausea and vomiting, gravel in the bladder, dropsy and suppressed urine. For piles it has been injected into the rectum. It has been said to soothe inflammation of the kidneys and bladder and that it is quieting to the stomach and nerves and has been used after an emetic to soothe the stomach.

SPEEDWELL: *Veronica officinalis.* Also Bird's Eye, Cat's Eye, Fluellin. As a tea this has been used on minor skin blemishes and for coughs and catarrh. It is similar in taste to Chinese teas but has none of the negative effects.

SPIKENARD: *Aralia racemosa.* Petty Morrel, Spignet. Because of its strength as an alterative, it has been used in rheumatic and uric acid disorders, as well as in some skin diseases.

SQUAW VINE: *Mitchella repens.* Sometimes called Checkerberry, Deerberry, Hive Vine, One-berry Leaves, Partridge Berry, Winterberry, White Clover. Alone, or in combination with red raspberry leaves, squaw vine has been used during pregnancy and is said to ease childbirth. With olive oil or cream it is reportedly a good bath for sore nipples. It is claimed to be a good and mild wash for sore eyes and has been given to children for this purpose. It is usually combined with equal parts of witch hazel leaves and raspberry leaves. As an injection for mild leucorrhea, dysentery and gonorrhea this has been given, and it has also been used for gravel, uterine and urinary troubles, female disorders, and to increase the menstrual flow.

SQUILL: *Urginea scilla.* Commonly known as Scilla. As an expectorant and to relieve irritated mucous membranes, squill has been taken for coughs and bronchial afflictions. A large dose of the herb is reported to be an emetic.

STRAWBERRY: *Fragaria vesca*. This is the common garden strawberry, and it is claimed that both the berries and leaves have medicinal properties. A tea of the leaves is a tasty, caffein-free substitute for the usual table tea and has been said to be a tonic for the entire system. It has also been said to be a stomach cleanser and useful for bowel troubles. Taken internally it reportedly helps eczema, diarrhea, and dysentery, and weakness of the intestines. It has also been used externally as a wash and as an enema. A gargle has been used for sore mouth and throat.

SUMACH: *Rhus glabrum*. Equal parts of sumach berries and bark, white pine bark, and slippery elm have been said to be effective for syphilis and gonorrhea. This tea is reportedly an excellent cleanser for the system and an aid for leucorrhea, scrofula and internal sores or wounds. A tea of sumach berries alone has been reported helpful in bowel complaints, fever and diabetes. They are also an emmenagogue, stimulating menstrual flow.

SUMMER SAVORY: *Satureja hortensis*. The carminative effects of this herb have reportedly made it valuable in wind colic. As a warm tea it is said to increase menstrual flow and to bring on suppressed menstruation. It has also been taken for colds and toothache, and is a popular condiment.

SUNDEW: *Drosera rotundifolia*. Sometimes called Dewplant, Flytrap. Because of its reported effect on dry, tickling coughs, this has been taken for whooping cough.

SUNFLOWER: *Helianthus annuus*. Also Marigold of Peru. The seeds of this plant contain 53% protein, making them an excellent meat substitute. They have been used for centuries as a medicine and a preventive, as well as a staple food. Reportedly pulmonary afflictions, snake bite, and dry hair have all been aided through application of the plant. And no part of the plant need go to waste: the leaves have been added to cattle and poultry feed, and the seeds themselves have been fed to chickens to increase laying; the stem fibers have been used by the Chinese in the manufacture of paper and silk; the pith of the stalk is so light that it is employed in the manufacture of life-saving equipment; the flowers make a color-fast dye; and any left-over part of the plant may be applied as a mulch or composted for an organic fertilizer rich in potash.

TANSY: *Tanacetum vulgare*. Commonly called Arbor Vitae, Hineheel, Yellow Cedar. Often grown by gardeners as an insect repellent, this has been used as a tonic for the stomach and bowels. It has reportedly been used for indigestion and to expel worms. Although this has been used for suppressed menstruation and female nervousness or hysteria, it should never be taken during pregnancy as it may cause a miscarriage. It is said to strengthen weak veins, and that an application of the herb, hot, soothes bruises, swellings, inflammations, and sore eyes. This remedy must be used with caution, as it is a narcotic and an overdose may be fatal.

THYME: *Thymus vulgaris.* This is the common garden plant and popular seasoning. Taken hot, it causes profuse perspiration and has been used for treating colds. As an antispasmodic, taken cold, it reportedly checks coughs, whooping cough, cramps, and other stomach ailments, including diarrhea. It is a nervine and emmenagogue.

TOAD FLAX: *Linaria vulgaris.* Common names are Butter and Eggs, Flaxweed, Pennywort. This has been used most often with other herbs in an ointment to treat skin diseases or piles. It is reportedly used in cases of jaundice and as a hepatic.

TORMENTIL: *Potentilla tormentilla.* Sometimes called Septfoil. This herbal tonic is an astringent, and has been used in diarrhea and as a gargle.

TURKEY CORN: *Corydalis formosa.* Also Choise Dieyltra, Squirrel Corn, Staggerweed, Wild Turkey Pea. This is reportedly an antisyphilitic and used for all skin diseases. Taken as a tea it is a tonic and an herbal astringent.

TURPENTINE: *Pinus palustris* or *Pinus maritima.*
This is a product formed naturally in the wood
of various conifers. Though it is dangerous to
take the oil internally, it is used in some pharmaceutical prescriptions and reportedly has
been applied externally for rheumatism and
pulmonary complaints, and sprains. With castor
oil, it is said to expel tapeworm. The vapor is
an irritant and provokes coughing, causing the
expulsion of phlegm which has been said to be
helpful in cases of bronchitis and pneumonia.

TWIN LEAF: *Jeffersonia diphylla.* Also Ground
Squirrel Pea, Helmet Pod, Rheumatism Root,
Yellow Root. Because of its effects as an antispasmodic and antirheumatic, this has been
claimed to be useful for neuralgia, cramps and
rheumatism. As a poultice it has been said that
it relieves pain and, in severe pain, should be
taken internally. It also has been used in cases
of syphilis and as a gargle for throat afflictions.

UVA URSI: *Arctostaphylos uva ursi.* Also Bearberry, Bear's Grape, Kinpikinn Ick, Mealberry,
Mountain Box, Mountain Cranberry, Sagck-
homi, Universe Vine, Wild Cranberry. This is
used a great deal in combination with other
herbs. Taken internally or as a douche it has
been said to be effective for female disorders
and gonorrhea. An infusion has been used in
diabetes, Bright's disease, dysentery, hemor-

rhoids, and discharges from the bladder. It has astringent, nephreticum, and tonic properties as well.

VALERIAN: *Valeriana officinalis.* Sometimes referred to as All Heal, Set Wall, Vandal Root. As a nervine and antispasmodic, this has been taken for hysterics and colic and to induce sleep. Taken hot, it is an emmenagogue. It has been said that it is mild enough to give to children for measles and scarlet fever, but in excessive doses may cause headache. It also is claimed to soothe ulcers in the stomach and to prevent fermentation and gas. Taken internally and applied externally at the same time it reportedly promotes the healing of pimples and sores. With licorice, raisins and anise seed it has been used for cough, shortness of breath, and to expectorate phlegm. It has also been used for bladder stones. Often it has been used with skullcap, mistletoe and vervain.

VERVAIN: *Verbena officinalis, Verbena hastata.* Also Simpler's Joy, Traveler's Joy, Wild Hyssop. As a powerful diaphoretic, this has been claimed to be effective against fevers, colds, whooping cough, pneumonia, and has been taken also for its expectorant property in asthma and ague. As an emmenagogue, it reportedly increases menstrual flow and will help other female troubles as well. It is also a vermifuge, and it is said to cause the expulsion of worms; a tonic for the entire system; and a vulnerary.

VIOLET: See Blue violet.

WAHOO: *Euonymus atropurpureus.* Also Arrow Wood, Bitter Ash, Burning Bush, Indian Root, Pegwood, Spindle Tree, and Strawberry Tree. This is a laxative and has been used for dyspepsia, dropsy, and fevers. It is claimed to be a better remedy than quinine for the same ailments.

WATERCRESS: *Nasturtium officinale.* This herb grows wild or cultivated in gently moving streams and may be eaten in salads as a vegetable. It is an excellent source of the B-Vitamin complex, as well as Vitamin C and several others, and also supplies many health-fortifying minerals. It is therefore an antiscorbutic and has been used to strengthen the bloodstream and serves as a stomachic.

WATERDOCK: *Rumex aquaticus.* Sometimes called Bloodwort or Red Dock. This herb is both an alterative and detergent and has been taken for skin diseases, sluggish liver, and, as a mouthwash, for ulcers. The powdered root is claimed to be a medicinal tooth cleaner.

WATER PEPPER: *Polygonum punctatum.* Sometimes called Smart Weed. Its astringent properties make water pepper reportedly valuable in any cases where tissues must be drawn together, such as coughs or colds. For scanty menstruation, it has been given hot as an emmenagogue; it is said to be helpful in uterine troubles, gravel in the bladder, bowel complaints, and kidney disorders. It has been used as an enema or a hot fermentation externally applied, or for erysipelas, as a cold water wash.

WHITE BRYONY: *Bryonia alba, Bryonia dioica.* Sometimes known as Bryonia, Bryonin, English Mandrake, European White Bryony, Mandragora, Wild Bryony. For a diuretic, it is said to have a soothing and cleansing action and to clear the lungs and bronchial tubes and remove excess fluids from the glands. It has therefore been used in cases of pleurisy, dropsy, bronchitis, coughs and influenza and pneumonia. It reportedly tends to reduce the swelling of glands (in tonsillitis) and inflammation, especially of the heart, caused by rheumatism or gout.

WHITE CLOVERS: See Clover, white.

WHITE OAK: *Quercus alba.* Also referred to as Tanner's Bark. Both the leaves and the bark of the white oak tree are used, the inner bark being the most potent part. It is said that a strong tea may be used internally and externally to remove varicose veins. This tea is also good as a douche for leucorrhea and other uterine troubles. It has been used as an enema for piles, hemorrhoids, or any rectal problem. It has also been taken to stop internal hemorrhages.

WHITE POND LILY: *Nymphaea odorata.* Also Cow Cabbage, Toad Lily, Water Cabbage, Water Lily. As a strong astringent the root of the water lily has been given for leucorrhea (both as a douche and internally), diarrhea, scrofula, bowel ailments; its reported effect on the mucous membranes and inflamed tissues makes it a popular home remedy for sore throat and gums, swellings, boils, ulcers and dropsy. It is said to be mild enough to be given to children for bowel troubles, and has also been used in kidney troubles, catarrh of the bladder, and irritation of the prostate. Applied to wounds and cuts, the leaves reportedly hasten healing.

WHITE WILLOW: *Salix alba*. Sometimes known as Withe, Withy. This bark has been used to reduce fever and chills. It is reported to have a good effect on stomach troubles and heartburn. A tea of the leaves and buds has been used in gangrene, and eczema, used both as a tea and applied directly. It is said to stop bleeding of wounds, nosebleed, and to serve as an eyewash, diuretic and for rheumatism and ague. It is reportedly more effective than quinine when used for the same purposes.

WILD ALUM ROOT: *Geranium maculatum*. Sometimes American Kino Root, American Tormentil, Cranesbill, Crowfoot, Geranium, Storksbill, Wild Dovefoot. The powerful astringency of this root makes it helpful, both internally and externally. It has been taken for cholera, dysentery, diarrhea, piles, chronic ulcers, or mucous discharges from any part of the body (also used for this with golden seal). It reportedly also stops hemorrhaging, bleeding wounds, nosebleed and excess menstruation. As a douche it has been used for uterine troubles and leucorrhea.

WILD CARROT: *Daucus carota*. See Carrot.

WILD CHERRY: *Prunus virginiana*. Sometimes called Black Cherry, Black Choke, Cabinet Cherry, Rub Cherry. As a tonic, the inner bark has been used to tone the system. It is said to loosen phlegm in the throat and chest, acting as a pectoral, and to be effective in relieving colds, grippe, tuberculosis and asthma. It also has been used in dyspepsia, fevers and high blood pressure.

WILD OREGON GRAPE: *Berberis aquifolium*. Also California Barberry, Holly-leaved Barberry, Mahonia. This has been said to be a blood purifier, helpful for skin diseases, uterine problems and liver and kidney troubles. It has also been used as a tonic and alterative, and is said to relieve rheumatism, leucorrhea and constipation.

WILD PLUM: The bark is claimed to be the "best remedy for asthma."

WILD YAM: *Dioscorea villosa*. Also China Root, Colic Root, Devil's Bones, Yuma. Because of its soothing, nervine effects, this has been used for any type of nervous excitement and for neuralgia. Taken during pregnancy (it may be combined with squaw vine) it reportedly relieves pain, allays nausea, and, with ginger, helps prevent miscarriage. It is said to be helpful in expelling gas from the bowels, for cholera, rheumatic pains, and afflictions of the liver. It is also an antispasmodic.

WINTERCRESS: *Barbarea vulgaris.* Also known as Yellow Rocket. This herb makes an excellent addition to any salad or the leaves and stems may be steamed and eaten as a vegetable. It has been used primarily as an anti-scorbutic.

WINTERGREEN: *Gaultheria procumbens.* Common names are Beerberry, Boxberry, Caudad tea, Checkerberry, Chink, Ed Pollom, Ground Berry, Grouse Berry, Hillberry, Ivory Plum, Mountain Tea, Partridge Berry, Redberry Tea, Spiceberry, Wax Cluster. This is a well-known, old-fashioned herb that has been used for colic and gas in the bowels. The oil is reportedly useful in liniments for swellings, boils, ulcers and inflammations. In small doses it is said to stimulate the heart, respiration and stomach. The tea has been used as a wash for sore eyes, a douche for leucorrhea, and a gargle for sore throat and mouth. It reportedly is sometimes taken for rheumatism, rheumatic fever, scrofula, skin diseases and any bladder problems.

WITCH HAZEL: *Hamamelis virginiana.* Common names are Hazel Nut, Pistachio, Snapping Hazel, Spotted Alder or Elder, Striped Elder, Tobacco Wood, Winter Bloom. Because of its astringent property, the bark or leaves of this plant are claimed to arrest excessive menstruation and hemorrhages. For piles, especially when they are bleeding, it is reportedly used in an enema; this, it is said, will allay dysentery or diarrhea. The same tea has been used as a douche, for leucorrhea and gonorrhea. As a poultice or wash, the same tea reportedly soothes sore eyes, inflammations, bed sores and piles.

WOOD BETONY: *Betonica officinalis*. Betony, Bishopswort, Louse Wort. This herb, taken with skullcap and Calamus Root, has been known for a hundred years for its excellent effect as a stomachic and its effectiveness for digestive disorders in general. It is said also to stimulate, mildly, the heart. It reportedly will relieve the pain of headaches, gout, neuralgia, colic, and other pains in the head and face. More effective than quinine, it has also been taken in jaundice, palsy, convulsions, dropsy, grippe, colds, consumption and nervous ailments. It is a vermifuge and has been used to cause worms to be expelled from the system.

WOOD SAGE: *Teucrium scorodonia*. Also Garlic Sage, Wood Germander. This is a tonic and has been used to promote the appetite. Externally has been applied, with chickweed, to sores, ulcers, swellings and boils to soothe and heal. In combination with ragwort and comfrey, wood sage has been used as a poultice for tumors. It reportedly will increase the flow of urine and menstrual flow, and has been taken for colds, fever, kidney and bladder problems, and palsy.

WOOD SANICLE: See Sanicle.

WOOD SORREL: *Oxalis acetosella.* Sometimes known as Cuckoo Sorrel, Allelujah. This has been given as a cooling medicine (it is a refrigerant) to reduce fevers. It has also been used with other diuretics in some urinary conditions.

WORMWOOD: *Artemisia absinthium.* Also Ajenjo, Old Woman. Applied as a fermentation, this has been used for rheumatism, swellings and sprains. The oil has been used in liniments that are used for sprains, bruises, lumbago, and so on. It reportedly may be taken internally for liver troubles, including jaundice, and intermittent fevers, diarrhea, and leucorrhea. It is claimed to be an excellent appetizer, and will act as a vermifuge.

YARROW: *Achillea millefolium.* Sometimes called Ladies' Mantle, Milifoil, Millefolium, Noble Yarrow, Nosebleed, Thousand Leaf. This has been used for lung hemorrhages, and, if taken early in a cold, reportedly will break it up. It is also a powerful febrifuge when taken hot and has been used for dyspepsia, scanty or suppressed urine, and mucous discharges from the bladder. It is said to have been used successfully for typhoid fever too, and in diabetes, and Bright's disease. For piles and hemorrhoids an enema has brought relief, as it seems to have an excellent effect on the mucous membranes. A douche of yarrow has been used for leucorrhea and other vaginal problems. It is claimed that an ointment will help to heal wounds, ulcers, and fistulas, and is helpful in measles, smallpox, and chickenpox. With elder flowers and peppermint in equal quantities it has been taken for influenza.

YELLOW DOCK: *Rumex crispus.* Also called Curled Dock, Garden Patience, Narrow Dock, Sour Dock. The root of this plant is depurative. As a detergent, it has been applied to leprosy, running ears, impetigo, itch and sores. It is used both in the form of a tea and an ointment. Its astringent quality makes it useful for such diseases as scrofula, glandular tumors, swellings, and syphilis. For glandular tumors and swellings it has been applied as a fermentation wrung from the hot tea.

YERBA SANTA: *Eriodictyon glutinosum.* Also Consumptive Weed, Gum Plant, Bear's Weed, Mountain Balm, Tar Weed. Because it is a tonic and an expectorant, invigorating the system and facilitating expectoration, this has been used in chronic bronchitis, laryngitis, and other lung troubles. It reportedly brings relief of rheumatism and reduces discharge from the nose. It is often an ingredient in asthma prescriptions.

YERBA MATE: See Paraguay tea.

BIBLIOGRAPHY

D. T. Atkinson, M.D., *Magic, Myth, and Medicine*, N.Y., Premier Books, 1956.

L.H. Bailey, *Standard Cyclopedia of Horticulture*, Macmillan Co.

S. A. Barrett, *Material Aspects of Pomo Culture*, Public Museum of Milwaukee, 1952.

W. H. Bates, M.D., *Better Eyesight Without Glasses*, N.Y., Henry Holt, 1940, 1943.

May Bethel, *The Healing Power of Herbs*.

E. H. Blair, *Indian Tribes of Upper Mississippi and Great Lakes Region*, Cleveland, 1911.

Neltje Blanchan, *Nature's Garden*, N.Y., 1900.

Nathaniel Lord Britton and Addison Brown, *Illustrated Flora of the Northern United States and Canada*, N.Y., 1913.

Gilbert E. Brooke, "Handbook, Tropical Medicine," *Hygiene and Parasitology*, 1908.

Fearing Burr, *Field and Garden Vegetables of America*, Boston, 1885.

Alphonse de Candolle, *Origin of Cultivated Plants*, N.Y., 1885.

George F. Carter, "Some Hopi Indian Foods," *The Herbarist*, Boston, 1946.

Linda Clark, *Get Well Naturally,* ARC Books, N.Y., 1971.

R. Swinburne Clymer, M.D., *Nature's Healing Agents,* Philadelphia, Pa., Dorance and Co., 1963.

Mrs. William Starr Dana, *How to Know the Wild Flowers,* Charles Scribners Sons, N.Y., 1898.

Adelle Davis, *Let's Eat Right to Keep Fit,* N.Y., Harcourt, Brace, 1954.

John E. Eichenlaub, M.D., *A Minnesota Doctor's Home Remedies for Common and Uncommon Ailments,* N.Y., Prentice Hall, 1960.

F. Ellingwood, M.D., *Materia Medica and Therapeutics,* Chicago, Ill., Medical Press, 1898.

Catharyn Elwood, *Feel Like a Million,* N.Y., Devin-Adair, 1954.

George B. Emerson, *A Report on the Trees and Shrubs Growing Naturally in the Forests of Massachusetts,* Boston, 1875.

William L. Esser, *Dictionary of Foods,* John's Island, S.C., 1947.

John Milton Fogg, *Weeds of Lawn and Garden,* Philadelphia, 1945.

Wilfred Funk, Inc., *Universal Standard Encyclopedia,* 1956, 1957.

Ada E. Georgia, *A Manual of Weeds,* N.Y., 1925.

John Gerard, *The Herball, or Generall Historie of Plantes,* London, 1597.

Melvin R. Gilmore, *Indian Lore and Indian Gardens,* Ithaca, N.Y., 1930.

Thomas Green, *Universal Herbal,* London, 1823.

A. R. Harding, *Ginseng and Other Medicinal Plants,* L. N. Fowler and Co.

Ben Charles Harris, *Eat the Weeds; Better Health with Culinary Herbs,* Boston, 1952; *Kitchen Medicines,* Barre, 1968.

Henry Hartshorne, *Household Cyclopedia,* Philadelphia, 1871.

Healthful Living Digest, Winnipeg, Manitoba, Canada.

W. A. Henderson, *Modern Domestic Cookery,* N.Y.

Rackham Holt, *George Washington Carver,* Doubleday and Co., N.Y., 1943.

Claudia V. James, *Herbs & the Fountain of Youth; That Old Green Magic,* Amrita Books.

Joseph M. Kadens, M.D., Ph.D., *Modern Encyclopedia of Herbs,* Parker.

Peter Kalm, *Travels of North America,* London, 1772.

Harriet L. Keeler, *Our Northern Shrubs,* N.Y., 1903.

H. E. Kirschner, M.D., *Nature's Healing Grasses,* Yucaipa, Calif., H. C. White Publishers, 1960.

Jethro Kloss, *Back to Eden,* Longview Publishing House.

Emmanuel and Decaisne J. Le Maout, *A General System of Botany,* trans. London, 1873.

John Lindley, *Flora Medica,* London, 1838.

Alice Lounsberry, *A Guide to the Trees,* N.Y., 1900.

Richard Lucas, *Common and Uncommon Uses of Herbs for Healthful Living,* Arco Publishing Co., Inc.

W. N. McCartney, M.D., *Fifty Years a Country Doctor,* N.Y., E. P. Dutton, 1938.

Oliver Perry Medsger, *Edible Wild Plants,* Macmillan Co., N.Y., 1939.

Joseph E. Meyer, *The Herbalist,* Indiana Botanic Gardens, 1934.

William Meyrick, *New Family Herbal,* London, 1740.

Mooney, James, and Olbrechts, *The Swimmer Manuscript,* Smithsonian Institution, Bureau of American Ethnology, Washington, D.C., 1932.

Walter C. Muenscher, *Weeds,* N.Y., 1935.

Dr. Nehru's reference to onions; *Electronic Medical Digest,* Special Ed., 1960.

New England Farmer, Boston, Vols. 1850-62.

Edward Palmer, *Food Products of the North American Indians,* U.S. Dept. of Agriculture, Annual Report, 1870.

John Parkinson, *Theatrum Botanicum, the Theater of Plantes,* London, 1640.

Maude Gridley Peterson, *How to Know Wild Fruits,* N.Y., 1905.

Ehrenfried Pfeiffer, *The Earth's Face and Human Destiny,* Rodale Press, Emmaus, Pa., 1947.

W. W. Ray, *Common Edible Mushrooms of Oklahoma,* Okla. Agricultural and Mechanical College, Stillwater, 1943.

Wilfred, W. Robbins and Francis Ramaley, *Plants Useful to Man,* Pa., 1933.

Julia E. Rogers, *The Tree Book,* Doubleday, Page, and Co., N.Y., 1905.

Eleanor Sinclair Rohde, *A Garden of Herbs,* Boston, 1936.

Charles F. Saunders, *Useful Wild Plants of the U.S. and Canada,* Robert M. McBride, N.Y., 1920.

R. Brooks Simpkins, *Visible Ray Therapy of the Eyes,* Health Science Press, Rustington Sussex.

Boris Sokoloff, M.D., *Civilized Diseases. You Can Cure Them,* N.Y., Howell Soskin, 1944; *Middle Age is What You Make It,* N.Y., Greystone Press, 1938.

Elizabeth Terry, "Quacks," *National Health Federation Bulletin,* April 1963.

Carlson Wade, *Natural and Folk Remedies,* Parker Publishing Co., Inc.

Heinrich Wallnöfer and Anna Von Rottauscher, *Chinese Folk Medicine,* Crown Publishers, Inc.

Harold Ward, *Herbal Manual,* L. N. Fowler and Co., Ltd.

Heber W. Youngken, *Textbook of Pharmacognosy,* Philadelphia, 1936.

INDEX